Praise for *The* Hot Mommy

"Alison has created an effective, user-friendly book for new moms wishing to lose their baby weight that is fun to read and easy to follow. She provides invaluable nutritional information, including a variety of food options to choose from, and better yet she teaches women how to break down a day of eating. Her enthusiasm comes off the page and is contagious as well as motivating."

—**Marla Solomon,** Certified Nurse Midwife

"Alison came into my life for a reason. It isn't often that someone will reach out and help another human being the way she helped me from start to finish. She has a true gift and valuable information to offer any new mother who wants to reclaim her body, achieve a high level of fitness, and boost her energy."

—**Ana Lazardi,** from the Foreword

"The Hot Mommy Next Door Program has transformed my eating lifestyle as well as my body. Alison's straightforward approach simplifies the 'mystery' of nutrition and exercise, allowing the busiest of moms to incorporate the guidelines into their daily routines and to achieve realistic results. Best of all, I never feel deprived eating five meals a day, and I always look forward to indulging in the glory of my cheat meal."

—**Millie McPherson,** mother of two

"Kudos to Alison Fadoul for her realistic approach to fitness! Her book has a plan that includes precisely what items to buy at a real, everyday-accessible grocery store. Also included is a basic guideline of what to put in your mouth without feeling deprived. That kind of common sense takes away my ingenious ability to make up excuses and helps me get on track. Most especially, the book addresses mind/body/spirit connection, which was key for me. Face it, every woman wants to look her best, and even though I have a chaotic schedule as a single mom, I now see hope. Alison's commitment to helping us avoid excuses while squeezing in a little 'me' time at the gym has been nothing short of a miracle."

—**Isabelle Leger,** mother of two

"After having kids, I found myself working out but was extremely discouraged that I was not seeing any results. Then I met Alison. With the help of Alison's simple guidelines, I have been able to make smart choices as to what I put into my mouth and to make my workouts count. I'm excited that I am finally making progress towards my goals."

—**Rosie Gonzalez,** mother of two

"I was always an avid gym goer, but I was missing basic nutrition knowledge. Alison's clear and user-friendly eating guidelines equipped me with the tools I needed to make the right choices and take control of my health. Changing my eating habits, in combination with making every workout count per Alison's exercise guidelines, enabled me to achieve my personal best body. I'm excited to say that I have a better body than before having children!"

—**Albania Macrae,** mother of two

The Hot Mommy Next Door

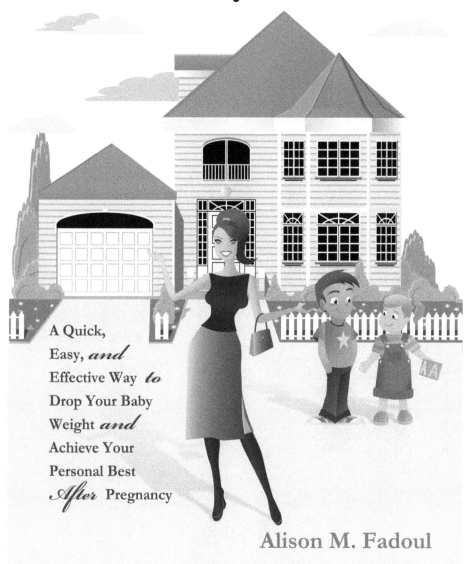

A Quick,
Easy, *and*
Effective Way *to*
Drop Your Baby
Weight *and*
Achieve Your
Personal Best
After Pregnancy

Alison M. Fadoul

New York

The Hot Mommy Next Door

By Alison M. Fadoul
© 2009 All rights reserved.

ISBN: 978-1-60037-554-5 (Paperback)

Library of Congress Control Number: 2008942181

Published by:

MORGAN · JAMES
THE ENTREPRENEURIAL PUBLISHER
www.morganjamespublishing.com

Morgan James Publishing, LLC
1225 Franklin Ave. Suite 325
Garden City, NY 11530-1693
800.485.4943
www.MorganJamesPublishing.com

Cover & Interior Designs:

Johnson2 Design

Megan Johnson
www.Johnson2Design.com

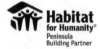

Habitat for Humanity®
Peninsula
Building Partner

In an effort to support local communities, raise awareness and funds, Morgan James Publishing donates one percent of all book sales for the life of each book to Habitat for Humanity.

Get involved today, visit:
www.HelpHabitatForHumanity.org

To my children, Mason and Morgan.
You have changed my life and my body forever.
May you always reach beyond your dreams,
as you have helped me realize mine.
I love you more than I can put into words.

Table *of* Contents

Acknowledgments

J would like to express my deep gratitude to my husband Charles, whose ongoing support and encouragement aided the completion of my book-writing journey. Now you can stop asking me when my book is going to be finished! Thank you for believing in me and in my dreams.

Thanks also to my mom, who always wanted to write a book and had the wit and humor to do so. I wrote one for both of us, Mom. I love you and feel your presence with me always.

A special thanks to my editor, Stephanie Gunning, who wore many hats during our journey together: my mentor, my confidante, my motivator, and best of all, my friend. I am still in awe that one person can know so much about so many different things. You have been a true inspiration.

Thanks to my friend Neki Mohan, whose wisdom, strength, and positive presence greatly influenced my determination to see this project through and whose referral to Laura Duksta led me to Sandy Grason and eventually to my favorite editor. Thanks to all of you for your part in bringing this project to fruition.

Thanks to all my friends and family for always believing in this project and me, especially when the fear got the better of me! To Ana Lazardi, my dear friend and sistah from anothah mothah, thanks for being my first guinea pig and my biggest fan. To Ana Baltar, my spiritual mentor, you helped me evolve and grow as a person over the course of our friendship. I know our paths' crossing was part of a bigger plan. And to Lily Valdivieso, my first personal trainer, thanks for showing me the ropes way back when. To all my fellow gym goers/moms/ friends/trainers/instructors thanks for your encouragement and motivation.

A special thanks to Marla Solomon, my nurse practitioner of twelve years, for your words of encouragement and support.

Thank you to Sheah Rarback, the Nutrition Division Director at the University of Miami, Miller School of Medicine, for taking the time to meet with me to discuss basic nutrition principles. Any factual errors that may remain in the book are my own.

I would also like to thank L.A. Fitness for allowing me the opportunity to share my passion of indoor cycling with their members on a weekly basis. And thanks to everyone who comes to class. (Don't forget to keep those abs tight and make it count.)

Finally, a heartfelt thanks to all of the women who stepped out of their comfort zone and made the effort to approach me with their fitness and health inquiries. You reinforced the message the universe was sending me to embark on this project. You have transformed my life, and I thank you.

Foreword

Ana Lazardi

*P*ick a diet, any diet ... and I bet you that I've tried it. You'd think that after the umpteenth unsuccessful diet maybe I would get a clue, but instead I continued to opt for fad diet after fad diet. Sure I would lose a couple of pounds for a couple of minutes, but the pounds always returned with a vengeance when I retired the diet and returned to my "normal" eating practices. Add two pregnancies within a year of each other to the mix, and you can see how I was easily left with more than a few unwelcome pounds, a body I did not recognize, and low self-esteem.

When a very pregnant mommy named Alison Fadoul walked her almost-three-year-old son into my classroom for the start of a new school year, I had no idea how much my life would be transformed and enriched by her presence. I'd all but given up on the idea that I'd ever succeed at getting rid of the weight I so desperately wanted to lose. In defeat, I didn't know where to turn for comfort other than the cookie jar, which of course only compounded the problem.

Then, during only a few short months after Alison gave birth to her daughter, I watched her go from a mom about to pop to one hot mama right before my eyes. Although I took note of her successful weight loss, I never thought that her fitness, eating, and lifestyle accomplishments could also be mine.

As weeks went by and my relationship with Alison slowly evolved from one of teacher and parent to a friendship, I became more forthcoming with her about my diet traumas. Alison always encouraged me and gave me fitness and healthy eating tips, but for a long time I didn't internalize her advice.

But one night over dinner, our conversation turned to dieting and body image. It was in this moment that my new, healthier life began. Alison told me that she was writing a book and could help me lose the weight I wanted to lose if I was seriously committed to myself and to the process. The next afternoon, Alison took me shopping and taught me the nutritional information that would provide the basis for my success. In less than two weeks, my scale registered ten pounds lighter, and I hadn't even stepped foot into a gym yet.

Fortunately, Alison insisted that a lifestyle of exercise combined with my new eating plan was a must. She even arranged a meeting for me with the manager of a nearby gym to see which trainer would suit my schedule. Six months later I was thirty-five pounds lighter, leaner, and feeling like a new woman. Since then I've kept the weight off, and I love how I feel. I believe I now look on the outside the way I've always felt on the inside—slim, beautiful, and athletic—and my energy has skyrocketed.

Alison came into my life for a reason. It isn't often that someone will reach out and help another human being the way she helped me. She has a true gift and valuable information to offer any new mother who wants to reclaim her body, achieve a high level of fitness, and boost her energy. With Alison's continued support and phenomenal guidance, I was able to realize that I could achieve my personal best. Her compassion for others, and her desire to help them feel good about themselves, has changed my life forever. Now I'm one hot mama, too—and if I can do it, so can you.

Introduction
Why I Wrote This Book

he book you're holding in your hands right now, *The Hot Mommy Next Door,* is a byproduct of the positive feedback I received for quickly getting back into shape after my second child was born. Lots of other moms acknowledged and praised my efforts. Their praise, of course, was always followed by the inquiry, *How* did you do it? They were eager to get in shape like me. I wanted to tell them how and to explain the steps in detail because I'm a Virgo, a woman, and a Type A personality, so I wrote a book. By sharing my story, hopefully I can touch, even transform, more women's lives than I could by telling people individually how I did what I did.

This book is written for moms from a mom's perspective because that's the real credential I have that merits writing this book. I'm a woman who went through two pregnancies and felt determined to get her body back as soon as possible. I'm not a celebrity. I'm just the mom next door with a story to tell.

Three years ago, after the birth of my daughter, I had a specific goal to transform my body and take my fitness to a higher level. I was blessed with two beautiful children and knew that a third pregnancy was not on my to-do list. So I was ready. I began to research what I would need to successfully reach my fitness goals. Everything I learned about health and taking care of my body is in this book.

How to Use This Book

By writing *The Hot Mommy Next Door,* I am hoping to pay forward to you the rewards I have received from others. I want to help you take charge of your fitness and feel good about your body. This book is designed to be a quick read so that you can get through it in one or two sittings after putting your kids down for a nap or to bed. You may also want to consult it regularly while on your journey to lose your "baby" weight and get back into shape. This book is your CliffsNotes (if you will) to a lifestyle that will help you get back into shape. As a mom with two young kids, I haven't read a whole book since I was on bed rest during my pregnancy with my first child. I bet you don't have much time to read either.

Here, you will find all the information you need to get started on your personal weight loss journey: Smart Choices Eating Guidelines; user-friendly menu options, complete with recipes and a detailed shopping list; goal-setting strategies; and clear instructions for getting into peak condition. To the best of my ability, I have adopted a straightforward approach to the subjects of basic nutrition, exercise, and self-discipline.

That being said, this one goes out to all you ladies!

Chapter 1

Two Kids, a Minivan, & No More Excuses

*A*t one point or another, we all ask ourselves, "Who am I?" When I first became a mom, this question took on a new level of importance for me. Before my son was born three and a half years ago, I couldn't answer it. But his birth put my life into perspective. In some regards, it was like undergoing my own rebirth. Finally I was able to define my identity and my goals to my own satisfaction. I was the happiest I'd ever been. Subsequently, after the birth of my daughter two years later, I gained more clarity and fine combed my answer. Unfortunately, I also gained weight. The good news was that the experience of two pregnancies and the resulting weight gain inspired me to take charge of my life and my fitness, and ultimately it inspired me to write this book. Everything I learned from my role as a mom about taking care of my body and health is in this book.

Now, you may be asking, "What is she babbling about and how does it pertain to me?" Well, let me fast forward a bit. After all, who has time to read a long book when you have young kids, right?

My commitment to fitness began after my first child was born. Prior to then, my workouts consisted of cardio classes here and there. If I did any weight training, it was a minimal leg workout done in an uninformed way. I never did an upper body workout unless it was part of one of the cardio classes I took. But my interest in fitness was different after the birth of my son. The physical changes and loss of control over my body that I had experienced during pregnancy weighed heavily on my mind (no pun intended ... okay, maybe a little pun intended). I was determined to lose my baby weight and then some.

After several months of going to the gym on a near-daily basis and casually monitoring my diet, my determination paid off, and I was successful in reaching my goal. I had gained forty-two pounds during my first pregnancy for a grand total of 172 pounds at delivery. I was twenty-eight years old and with a modest degree of commitment and effort, I managed to lose fifty-four pounds, bringing me three pounds shy of my weight at age twenty-one. Because I stand a petite 5'4" in my socks, 118 pounds is an appropriate and healthy weight for me.

Today, I attribute that first successful post-pregnancy weight loss to learning formal weight training practices and to increasing the number of cardiovascular workouts I was doing. Yes, I watched what I ate, but only to a degree. The truth is that I was more liberal then than now in the choices that I made about what I put in my mouth, primarily due to a lack of knowledge. My thought process was that small indulgences didn't matter when actually they add up. I treated myself to dessert nightly with an ice cream marketed as a "healthier choice." Although it was low fat, it had tons of sugar in it. I was happy with my results but knew I planned to get pregnant again, so I intentionally didn't take my fitness goals and exercise regimen to the next level.

Skip ahead to the birth of my second child. My baby girl arrived by cesarean section, so I was forced to wait and heal from the surgery before heading to the gym. By the time it was allowed, I was chomping at the bit to get back into shape.

Lord knows I had grown tired of seeing the beautifully shaped bodies at my gym while my body continued to expand with every passing day of my pregnancy. Toward the end of my pregnancy, my trips to the gym were just a formality. Right after the birth, I had to give myself a chance to recover from the surgery and stitches. But I hit the gym as soon as I had my six-week post-baby checkup with the doctor. (Okay, I'm lying. It was actually five days before my six-week appointment with the obstetrician was scheduled.) Remember, it is safest and most prudent to ask your doctor before resuming strenuous physical activity.

Still struggling with the aches and pains from the C-section I'd had, I slowly got back into the swing of things. Regaining control of my body and life made me feel like a new woman. Now I was on a mission to take my body to a higher level of fitness than I'd ever achieved before, and I wanted to see how quickly—yet safely—I could accomplish that goal.

Other moms repeatedly told me how hard it was to get back into shape after their second child, especially once they hit thirty (I was then thirty-one, thank you). But I really must thank those moms because they scared me into shape. In only three months—using the exact same eating guidelines and exercise regimen that I spell out in this book—I got back to my prepregnancy weight of 118. A month after that, I was another six pounds lighter, leaner, and better defined. I won't lie that it took some effort.

The idea to write a book sharing a realistic post-pregnancy weight loss and fitness plan came to me at the gym in the middle of a routine workout when yet another observer praised the results of my efforts and commented that I did not look like a mom of two kids. To which I thought, *What does a mom of two kids look like?* Why shouldn't we equate moms with fitness? I already had a minivan to identify my momness. I didn't need leftover pregnancy weight to reveal my status!

Two Kids, a Minivan, and No More Excuses

How sad is it that women are almost expected to have a permanently altered body after having a baby? Is having a baby supposed to be like a Community Chest card in the game Monopoly? "Had a baby. Ten extra pounds of weight forgiven and expected. Go straight to the nearest sweetshop." Recent pregnancy is a perfect excuse for any extra pounds that are hanging around. It is so easy just to let go and give up on your body.

In reality, with some effort and by making good choices about what you put in your mouth and how frequently you exercise, you can drop the baby weight. You've got to be honest with yourself about the choices you are making if you have any hope of success. True. Your body is never quite the same after pregnancy, but your personal best is still attainable. I promise!

It seems that everywhere I go these days, from the drycleaner to the local day spa, I receive a great response to the effort I've made to get back into shape quickly. The women I talk to seem to think I have a highly guarded secret. New moms and veteran moms alike have approached me to ask how I lost weight and got fit. Future moms have told me how much they hope to be in similar shape after having their own kids. "What is your secret?" they ask. "What do you eat? How do you train?" No matter with whom I am speaking, I always answer the same way, "There is no secret. You, too, can be in the incredible shape you want to be in."

One time when my daughter was four months old, I recall how I ran into a woman at the gym who felt compelled to ask my daughter's age. She openly gave my body the once-over. As a woman, I knew exactly what she was doing. Who are we fooling? Women all check each other out! As I answered the woman's initial question, I could see her brain processing the information that my daughter was four months old and trying to reconcile it with the fit condition of my body. Intrigued, she then proceeded to ask me a series of specific questions. How did I get back into shape so quickly, what did I eat or not eat, and so on?

The good news is there is no secret. Nonetheless, moms with young kids and infants need simple, clear information on how to get into shape due to the time demands of raising children. As moms, we all look and listen to one an-other regarding the latest stages in our children's development. We ask, "How did you get your baby to sleep through the night? How many times a day do you feed your baby solids," and so on? I think it's high time that we also look to one another for advice regarding our own physical well-being.

That said, it is important for us to stop comparing our bodies to those of other women and to learn to do what is right for us. Fitness and health ulti-mately influence every other part of our lives. As my mom always told me, "If you look good, you'll feel good and you'll do good." From my own experi-ence, I concur. Truly, I am a better mom because I take time out of each day to take care of myself. This is a physical, emotional, and mental necessity.

Part of the reason I've received such an overwhelmingly positive and vo-cal response to my appearance is that other moms identify with me. We share similar lives. I am your average stay-at-home mom with two kids, sporting around town in my minivan (yes, I surrendered and got one even though I swore I never would). I'm neither a professional athlete nor a personal trainer. Nor do I belong to the financial elite who has meals from The Zone diet deliv-ered to their doorsteps and keep personal trainers on retainer. I am a normal person who has achieved realistic results with a little bit of knowledge, deter-mination, hard work, commitment, and desire.

During my adult life, even when I was not pregnant, my body weight has ranged from 130 pounds at my heaviest to 106 pounds at my lightest (when I was eighteen). Sometimes I felt good about myself, sometimes not so much. I know what it feels like not to be happy with the shape you're in.

Low self-esteem can create a vicious cycle that leads to poor fitness. I know this cycle all too well: You're depressed about the way you look, so you eat. Then you figure, what's the point of going to the gym? You have such a long way to go to get to where you want to be and wonder if your body is capable of looking the way you fantasize about it looking anyhow. So you give up.

Two Kids, a Minivan, and No More Excuses

It is hard to climb up the hill of fitness, but once you're at the top, the view is worth it and it's not as hard to stay there. If you truly want the body you've always wanted, you'll put your cross-trainers on and drag your sorry butt up that damn hill.

Ladies, it is called a *workout* for a reason. It is hard work. But anything worth having is worth working for, right? Your personal best is in your reach. You just have to reach out and make it happen. No more excuses! From this day forward, you must decide what shape you are in by virtue of the choices you make.

The Hot Mommy Next Door

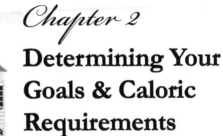

Chapter 2

Determining Your Goals & Caloric Requirements

*T*he first step to achieving your goals is to define them. You need to ask yourself what exactly you want to accomplish at the gym and with your eating plan. Then you must figure out how many calories you need to eat on a daily basis to reach your goals. How low can that number drop without sacrificing your health? Many different factors affect your caloric requirements: your height and weight, your level of activity, and if you are breastfeeding.

Let's begin by discussing the goal-setting process.

Defining Your Goals

I made great personal progress at the gym after my first baby was born. I had packed on forty-two pounds and was able to lose fifty-four for a final weight of 118, several pounds lighter than my prepregnancy weight. But I lost control of my weight again due to my second pregnancy. Knowing I was finished having babies after my second child was born, I decided to take my body to the next level. My personal goal was to have a body that was long, lean, and cut.

Originally I wanted my body to look like that of a woman who trains to compete in fitness competitions, although I was not actually interested in competitions. As I started to see the positive results of my workouts and became more informed, however, I realized that to look like a professional fitness competitor was a full-time job. That was unrealistic for my personal lifestyle as the stay-at-home mom of two small children, and so I happily modified my goals. You, too, will more than likely modify your goals as you make progress toward them. Ultimately, my goal was to appear athletic enough that people could tell by looking at me that I worked out.

In defining your fitness goals, a good place to start is to assess your physical condition at six weeks postpartum, the time when most women's doctors give them the green light to resume normal activity and exercise. While we're on the subject of doctors, please consult your doctor before heading to the gym for the first time after having a baby, especially if you had any kind of surgery. You're going to be working out hard, and you need to be sure it's safe.

Unfortunately, at this point you may not recognize the body attached to you below your neck. After my pregnancy, I personally tried not to look down too often. I figured that what I didn't know couldn't scare the heck out of me. Although I was aware that there was a jelly belly down there, I had decided not to acknowledge its presence.

So, take a moment now to introduce yourself to your temporarily altered, post-baby body. But tell it not to get too comfortable because it won't be there for long. You're going to work it off.

Following Baby number two, I made it a point not to step on a scale until my sixth week postpartum visit to my ob-gyn. I'll never forget that dreaded weigh-in. Even though I'd been careful to eat well since the birth, and I knew that I'd dropped quite a bit of weight already, staring me straight in the face was the reality of weighing 130 pounds. This meant I still had another whopping twelve pounds to lose to get back to my prepregnancy weight of 118.

With my doctor's permission, I slowly headed back to the gym on a daily basis to reacquaint my body with the degree of weight training and cardiovascular activity that it had not seen since I was seven and a half months pregnant. Just taking the step to improve my physical condition was empowering.

It felt great to be back at the gym. However, I will never forget my first jog on the treadmill on my first day back. After ten minutes or so my body itched all over from the long-unfelt sensation of blood circulating, and I felt as though my insides were being shifted out of place with every step. I knew I had a challenging uphill road ahead of me but there would be no turning back. My sights were set on my goal (long, lean, and cut) and I was hell bent on reaching it.

Do you have a picture in mind of how you'd like to look? Write it down here. "I'd like to look: _____
_____."

Body Composition Analysis

The first step to take toward your new body is to have a body composition analysis completed at a gym. Perhaps you belong to a gym or plan to join one in the near future. If so, this test is a simple request. It may be free to members or you may be charged a small fee for this service. Frequently, it is included as part of a gym package, especially if you hire a trainer or are just taking out a membership. If you'll be working out in your home, make a trip to the nearest gym and pay the small fee to have the test completed. You may also opt to purchase your own scale, which will allow you to continue to track your progress toward your goals.

Determining Your Goals & Caloric Requirements

A body composition analysis is simple, painless, and takes only a couple of minutes to complete. It involves standing barefoot on a special scale that accounts for your height, weight, age, and gender. According to Tanita, the world leader in precision electronic scales, through a process called Bioelectrical Impedance Analysis (BIA), electrodes in the scale's foot sensor pads send a low, safe signal through the body. "BIA measures the impedance or resistance to the signal as it travels through the water that is found in muscle and fat."[1] Honestly, the hardest part of this test is being asked to divulge your age!

A trainer may also measure your body composition with a tool called a skin-fold caliper, with which he or she gently pinches your flesh at specific body sites.

A third method, which is more complicated but the most accurate, involves dunking you in a tank of water. This process, known as hydrostatic weighing, involves submerging a motionless, minimally-clothed individual under water, once she has expelled all of the air from her lungs. Hydrostatic weighing determines body fat percentage from body density, because muscle and fat have different densities.

Simply put, body composition analysis tells you how much of your current weight is made up of fat and how much of your weight is made up of muscle. A personal trainer or nutritionist can help you translate that information into how many calories per day you should intake to maintain or lose weight. This will be your starting point of reference for your subsequent goals.

In the beginning, you should have your body composition analyzed at one-month intervals. It can be a real confidence booster to see your hard work paying off, as you swiftly make progress toward your goals. Most women who follow these guidelines drop significant weight in the first month. Their bodies react very positively when they switch to healthier foods and exercise regularly.

By the way, most women's body weight fluctuates according to their menstrual cycles. You'll probably be at your lowest weight somewhere in the middle of your cycle and at your heaviest weight just prior to getting your period. Furthermore, you'll weigh less first thing in the morning before eating or drinking anything. So if you want a psychological lift, get your body composition analysis done early in the day sometime midmonth.

What does a second body composition analysis tell you? You might find when you're tested that, although you've dropped pounds, you still have a higher ratio of fat to muscle than you'd like. Or perhaps you'll find that although your weight did not drop, you converted some of your fat to muscle for a lower percentage of body fat. Remember, muscle weighs more than fat! You might discover that you are ready to change from an eating plan for weight loss to an eating plan for weight maintenance. No matter what you find, use the information as a source of motivation to continue working toward your fitness goals.

Body Mass Index

Another way to assess your condition, albeit less accurate than a body composition analysis, is by determining your body mass. The Body Mass Index (BMI) is a measure of body fat that evaluates weight in relation to height. This tool tells you if you are at a healthy weight or are at possible risk for weight-related problems such as diabetes or high blood pressure. It is important to note, however, that BMI is only one factor related to risk for disease.

BMI is not a direct measure of body fat because it is calculated from an individual's weight, which includes both muscle and fat. However, according to the U.S. Centers for Disease Control (CDC), BMI is a generally reliable indicator of percentage of body fat. A BMI of 30 or greater is considered obese, a BMI of 25–29.9 is considered overweight, and a BMI of 18.5–24.9 is considered normal. Any BMI percentage below that is considered underweight.[2] As your fitness level improves, tracking your BMI may be good for your confidence and may boost your motivation.

Determining Your Goals & Caloric Requirements

Use the table below to calculate your BMI. To use the table, find your height in the left-hand column. Move across the row to find your weight. The number at the top of the column is the BMI for that height and weight.

Body Mass Index Table

BMI	19	20	21	22	23	24	25	26	27	28	29	30	31	32	33	34	35	36	37	38
Height (Inches)									Body Weight (Pounds)											
60	97	102	107	112	118	123	128	133	138	143	148	153	158	163	168	174	179	184	189	194
61	100	106	111	116	122	127	132	137	143	148	153	158	164	169	174	180	185	190	195	201
62	104	109	115	120	126	131	136	142	147	153	158	164	169	175	180	186	191	196	202	207
63	107	113	118	124	130	135	141	146	152	158	163	169	175	180	186	191	197	203	208	214
64	110	116	122	128	134	140	145	151	157	163	169	174	180	186	192	197	204	209	215	221
65	114	120	126	132	138	144	150	156	162	168	174	180	186	192	198	204	210	216	222	228
66	118	124	130	136	142	148	155	161	167	173	179	186	192	198	204	210	216	223	229	235
67	121	127	134	140	146	153	159	166	172	178	185	191	198	204	211	217	223	230	236	242
68	125	131	138	144	151	158	164	171	177	184	190	197	203	210	216	223	230	236	243	249
69	128	135	142	149	155	162	169	176	182	189	196	203	209	216	223	230	236	243	250	257
70	132	139	146	153	160	167	174	181	188	195	202	209	216	222	229	236	243	250	257	264
71	136	143	150	157	165	172	179	186	193	200	208	215	222	229	236	243	250	257	265	272
72	140	147	154	162	169	177	184	191	199	206	213	221	228	235	242	250	258	265	272	279

Source: National Heart Lung and Blood Institute, adapted from Clinical Guidelines on the Identification, Evaluation, and Treatment of Overweight and Obesity in Adults: The Evidence Report.[3]

Setting Your Goals

Three months after giving birth to my daughter, I hired a personal trainer who did my first body composition analysis. At that point I had lost ten of the twelve pounds I had decided to lose and was down to 120 pounds, two pounds shy of my original goal to reach my prepregnancy weight of 118. That was exciting news. But it wasn't the end. I still wanted to be lean and have well-defined muscles.

The new information I received was that my body fat was at 24.5 percent, which is average, meaning neither good nor bad. It felt like I was receiving a report card for my body in the neighborhood of a B when I really wanted to get an A+.

People often say that what you don't know won't hurt you. In this case, however, what you *do* know will empower you! To see this information on paper made it real to me and helped me face facts. I knew I had to keep going until I lowered my body fat. If your body composition numbers indicate you are within the lower spectrum of the normal range, congratulations. Keep doing whatever you're doing in the gym and keep eating well.

If your body composition numbers indicate that you are average, like I was, perhaps that will give you the incentive you've needed to strive to be better than average.

If your body composition analysis indicates you are overweight (or even obese) based upon your weight and the percentage of your body fat, I hope it jump-starts you into action. Don't beat yourself up. Just get moving. Use the eating and exercise guidelines that worked for me.

Upon learning the makeup of my body, I set a new goal for myself. It was time to get lean and cut. My trainer said I could set a goal to have between 14 and 17 percent of body fat without being unhealthy if I was careful to receive adequate nutrition. We discussed the feasibility of reducing another five pounds of weight so I'd get down to 115. But my trainer indicated that my body might be "happy" at 120 pounds. Everyone has a point at which she

Determining Your Goals & Caloric Requirements

functions optimally. However, my trainer also said it would be possible for me to convert more fat pounds into muscle.

We discussed my eating habits, which I subsequently tracked in a journal for a few days for my trainer's review. Looking over my notes she was able to inform me of the changes I needed to make to see the results that I so desired. One month later, I was another six pounds lighter and leaner. I'd reached a lovely 114, which eventually—with continued hard work—became 109 pounds and 15.2 percent body fat, a weight and body composition I have maintained since then.

This experience, my friends, was where my new life began and was the source of inspiration for The Hot Mommy Next Door Program. Not only did I become more fit, in the process I developed a love of exercise and ultimately became a certified SPIN® instructor, teaching classes regularly at my local gym.

After gaining baby weight, a realistic first goal for most moms is to strive for their prepregnancy weight. Since you have been there before it is a safe bet that you can get there again. You may be thrilled with that achievement and decide to maintain that weight forever.

Of course, you may want to set a new and different goal. Perhaps your prepregnancy weight was more than you previously weighed and you'd like to set a new goal to aim for that previous weight. Maybe you would like to see some definition in your muscles. Our goals are all different. The main goal is to be the best you that *you* can be.

As you are starting out, be flexible in your goals. Aim for the stars but be willing to adjust your goals according to your lifestyle and your body. Please don't compare yourself to others because you can set yourself up for failure. And please, please don't compare your body to the body of a twenty-something woman who has no kids, because that type of comparison could send you right over the edge.

And remember always to consult your doctor or health-care provider before heading to the gym, especially if the only weight you have ever picked up is you getting out of bed or reaching for a two-liter bottle of Diet Coke in the pantry.

If you have very recently had a baby, whether by vaginal birth or caesarean section, you must listen to the signals of your body. It will tell you when you are pushing yourself too hard and are in need of rest. It is essential to slowly build up your strength and modify your workout to fit your current abilities.

Daily Caloric Requirements

You must know your body in order to help your body. This is where interpreting your body composition analysis comes into play. Your analysis indicates what your caloric intake should be based on your percentage of body fat and weight. By utilizing the above three factors, you can determine your basal metabolic rate (BMR), which is the number of calories you would expend if you did zero activity on a given day. Once you determine your BMR, you must then factor in your daily activity in order to calculate your daily caloric expenditure.

The International Sports Science Association (ISSA) gives an easy four-step mathematical formula for calculating BMR once you know your percentage of body fat, as you will if you've done a body composition analysis or read the BMI table (see p. 14). I have adapted their formula for this text.[4] For the sake of example, let's pretend you weigh 172 pounds, are 5'6" tall, and have 24.5% body fat.

STEP *1*:

For this formula to work, you must convert your weight from pounds (lbs) into kilograms (kg). To do so, divide your weight by 2.2.

Example: 172 lbs ÷ 2.2 = 78.18 kg

Now do yours: _____

Determining Your Goals & Caloric Requirements

STEP 2:

Multiply your weight in kilograms by 0.9 and then by 24. Round off to the nearest whole number.

Example: 78.18 x 0.9 x 24 = 1,689

Now do yours: _____

STEP 3:

Use the table below to identify your personal multiplier based on the body fat percentage you previously determined through your body composition analysis at the gym (see page 11) or by referring to the BMI table (see page 14).

Percent Body Fat	Multiplier
Women 14 to 18%	1.00
Women 18 to 28%	0.95
Women 28 to 38%	0.90
Women over 38%	0.85

Then multiply your total from Step 2 by your personal multiplier. The resulting figure is your Basal Metabolic Rate (BMR). Round off to the nearest whole number.

Example: 1,689 x 0.95 (based on a body fat of 24.5%) = 1,605 calories

Now do yours: _____

Remember, this number is representative of the amount of calories you would expend doing no activity during the day.

STEP 4:

Identify your activity level from the following list of descriptions, to determine your activity multiplier.

Activity Level	Multiplier
No exercise	1.30 (130%)
Light activity: some walking throughout the day	1.55 (155%)
Moderate activity: walking, jogging, gardening, cycling, tennis, dancing, skiing or weight training 1–2 hours per day	1.65 (165%)
Heavy Activity: manual labor, such as digging, tree felling, climbing, or 2–4 hours of sports per day (football, soccer, or body building)	1.80 (180%)
Very Heavy Activity: a combination of moderate and heavy activity for 8 or more hours per day, plus 2–4 hours of intense training per day	2.00 (200%)

Then, multiply your BMR by your activity multiplier to determine your total daily caloric expenditure.

Example: 1,605 x 1.55 (light activity) = 2,488 cal.

Now do yours: _____

Breastfeeding Moms and Weight Loss

The good news for most women is that breastfeeding increases total daily caloric expenditure. Breastfeeding is an easy, natural way to burn five to six hundred calories a day without even trying. According to La Leche League International, mothers who choose to breastfeed should wait at least two months postpartum to lose weight purposefully, due to the time that is needed to recover from childbirth and establish a good milk supply.

Determining Your Goals & Caloric Requirements

After the two-month postpartum mark, La Leche League recommends a gradual weight loss of one pound per week. It is no surprise that they also suggest consulting your physician before starting a weight loss program while breastfeeding. That's because your baby's need for adequate nutrition must supersede all other goals you may have concerning food. Babies that are undernourished fail to thrive.[5]

So go ahead and ask your pediatrician, postpartum doula, or other health care provider a lot of questions about your meals especially if your baby isn't gaining as much weight as hoped. But if your breastfed baby is thriving and you've been given a green light to begin weight loss, move forward confidently. It should be a smidgen easier for you to lose weight in the beginning.

Putting This Information to Work for You

Let's assume that your primary fitness goal after pregnancy is to lose your baby weight. To do that, you'll need to take in fewer calories than you burn per day. Every 3,500 calories is equivalent to one pound. So in order to lose one pound of fat per week, you would need to make sure you consume 3,500 calories less per week than you expend or 500 calories less per day than you expend. That's why you need to know your total daily caloric requirement to be successful.

Three months after giving birth my total daily caloric requirement if I wanted to maintain my weight was 1,846 calories. For a planned weight loss of 1 pound per week, here's the math: 1,846 calories minus 500 calories per day allowed me a total caloric intake of 1,346 calories per day.

What if you calculated that you could consume 2,000 calories per day to maintain your weight? And let's just say, for the sake of an example, that you weren't an avid exerciser before pregnancy, let alone during pregnancy. By merely cutting back 500 calories a day to a 1,500 daily caloric intake and combining that with daily exercise periods—during which you burn a hypothetical 500 calories per day—you can expect your efforts to result in a two-pound per week weight loss.

Once you've dropped twenty or thirty pounds, you'll utilize the same BMR-based formula to determine again how many calories to consume in order to achieve and ultimately maintain your new weight. Your caloric intake should not be reduced more than the level required to maintain your weight at a desired level.

Does all of this seem confusing to you? Fortunately, there are professionals available to help you determine your true caloric needs. You may choose to consult a nutritionist or a personal trainer. That being said, a main purpose behind this program is to empower you with knowledge so you can begin to lose weight safely on your own.

Ladies, let's get clear right now about one thing: The Hot Mommy Next Door Program is not a diet. I repeat, this is *not* a diet.

"Why?" you might ask.

Well, I'll tell you: because diets don't last.

No, my friends, approach this as a *lifestyle*, a way of living healthy and eating healthy for the long run.

Imagine that your body is a machine. In order to function at its highest level, you must take in a certain amount of calories, or raw energy, every day as fuel. (We're not yet talking about the nutritional values of different foods.) If you do not consume the necessary amount of calories, your body recognizes the deficit, slows down your metabolism, and stores some of what you have eaten as fat. Fat is your body's reserve energy source. Your body is programmed to avoid starvation.

You do not need to starve yourself to lose weight, quite the contrary. In fact, if you consume the necessary amount of calories, your body burns what it needs to and processes the calories accordingly. This enhances your metabolism.

Determining Your Goals & Caloric Requirements

Eating many small meals a day, as you'll learn to do with these guidelines, contributes to boosting your metabolism because your body thinks "Hey! I can use some of this for fuel, *and* I do not need to store the rest because I know that in a couple of hours my mouth will partake of another nutritious meal."

Once you have the necessary information regarding the caloric intake you need to reach your goals, you can begin to make the smart choices necessary to achieve your goal weight and physique. Spreading your caloric intake over five small meals throughout the day will leave you satisfied while also boosting your metabolism. That's always a plus!

Ultimately, you can achieve your desired results if you are truly committed to your health. If you understand the basics of what you are doing and why you are doing it, you can change your lifestyle and stay the course. You only have one body. If you take care of it, it will take care of you.

Eating is the key. I cannot stress this enough. Even if you spend an hour at the gym on a daily basis there are still twenty-three hours left in a day to fall off the health wagon. You must know what caloric intake your body needs to make your goals a reality as well as what the right things to eat are. Then you can eat to live rather than live to eat.

Are you ready and excited to learn the details of eating well so that you can regain your fitness and be the best *you* in the future? Then turn the page and read on.

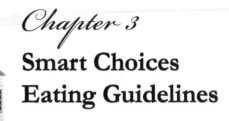

Chapter 3

Smart Choices
Eating Guidelines

*T*he good news, ladies, is that there are no real secrets to weight loss and fitness. Your common sense combined with a little nutritional guidance will go a long way. That's why the heart of the Hot Mommy Next Door Program is so easy to grasp and use. It is designed to fit the on-the-go lifestyle of a mom with young children. In this chapter, you'll learn what to eat, when to eat, and how to eat to achieve the best you safely and swiftly.

In a nutshell, here are the five basic principles of the Smart Choices Eating Guidelines:

1. Eat five small, well-balanced meals a day: three main meals and two healthy snacks. Divide your caloric and nutritional requirements among them.

2. Eat two and a half to three and a half hours apart. Three hours is ideal, but as moms we don't always get to dictate our schedules precisely the way we'd like.

3. Eat "clean" meals consisting of lean protein, healthy fat, complex carbs, low sodium, and low to no sugar.

4. Drink eight to ten 8-ounce glasses of water at a minimum, and more when you exercise.

5. Enjoy one "cheat meal" each week.

That doesn't sound so hard, does it?

We all put certain foods in our mouths that we know won't enhance our figures. Think french fries, think chocolate, think french fries dipped in a chocolate milkshake (okay, that's enough … quit thinking!) Perhaps identifying the wrong things to eat is a bit easier than identifying the right things to eat. If there is a secret to eating to achieve peak fitness and maintain a high-energy lifestyle, the secret is making sense of nutritional information recommended by various sources. Unless you are a nutritionist, chances are you need a little help in this area. While I am not a professional nutritionist, I have done research to formulate these eating guidelines and have consulted Sheah Rarback, the Nutrition Division Director at the University of Miami Miller School of Medicine.

Some people have the misconception that if they work out they can eat whatever and whenever they want. Two words, ladies: not so! Only a few genetically blessed women can get away with that philosophy. At each meal you must feed your body only what it needs and can utilize in the short-term. Your body will store anything else as fat.

The best news is that deciding to make smart choices limits the amount of options available. In essence, this makes it easier to stick to smart, healthy choices. If you follow the eating guidelines exactly and get regular exercise, you'll boost your metabolism, burn fat, and reduce weight. Then your confidence will grow.

The discipline and structure provided by eating five "clean" meals a day will improve your ability to succeed. And even if you find that you miss some foods you used to eat, once your brain and palate are retrained, you'll find most items in the guidelines delicious. Or save your favorite "sinful" foods for cheat meals—we'll talk more about that later in the chapter.

Decide to Eat "Clean"

In this program, you'll learn to eat clean. Eating clean entails choosing sources of lean protein, complex carbohydrates, healthy fats, and whole fruits. A major part of eating clean is eating low-sugar (or no-sugar) and low-sodium meals. By the time you finish this book, your new best friends will be the nutrition fact labels on products. Believe me, you'll see them in a whole new light.

Actually, you will see the entire grocery store in a whole new light. Almost every food in the Smart Choices Eating Guidelines can be found on the outskirts of most stores, because foods displayed in the aisles are bad news, except for a few items that we'll discuss later.

Before we talk about shopping, it's critical for you to understand that fats, carbohydrates, and proteins are all important elements in a healthy eating regimen. None of them should be eliminated. The key is to know which fats, carbohydrates, and proteins to consume in order to achieve the body you desire. You must also know *when* to eat the right fats, carbohydrates, and proteins.

Okay, ladies. Let's get down to business.

Smart Choices Eating Guidelines

Choose Healthy Fats

Healthy fats are unsaturated fats. They are essential for vitamin absorption and to maintain a healthy immune system. Unsaturated fats, also known as monounsaturated and polyunsaturated fats, may help to reduce blood cholesterol levels when used in place of saturated and trans fats.[6]

As with everything else in life, consume healthy fats responsibly—and by that I mean in moderation.

SOURCES OF HEALTHY FATS

Avocados, most nuts (peanuts, almonds, cashews, walnuts), seeds (sunflower, sesame), peanut butter, vegetable oils (olive oil, peanut oil, canola oil, safflower oil, sunflower oil, soybean oil, and cottonseed oil), cold-water fish (salmon, mackerel, trout), flaxseeds, and flax oil.

Beware of Bad Fats

Bad fats are comprised of saturated fats (found mostly in animal products) and trans fats (found primarily in fried and processed foods). Trans fats, although unsaturated, have a dual impact in that they can raise bad cholesterol and lower good cholesterol. According to the American Heart Association, the body typically makes all the cholesterol it needs. Therefore, it is not necessary to consume it.[7] Both types of bad fat can raise your blood cholesterol levels, thus increasing your risk of heart disease.[8]

When consuming products that contain saturated fats, such as cheese, stick to the low-fat or no-fat varieties and make sure to watch your serving size as much as humanly possible. Consume cheese cautiously to obtain the essential nutrients it contains, such as calcium.

I suggest you read the ingredient labels rather than the advertising promises when selecting products. For example, in the case of trans fats a company may label their product as containing 0 trans fats if the product contains less than 0.5 percent trans fats. I am grateful to Sheah Rarback, the Nutrition Division Director at the University of Miami, Miller School of Medicine for pointing out this little regulatory loophole. So beware. Make sure to skim the ingredients for the terms "hydrogenated" or "partially hydrogenated," and avoid them at all costs.

SOURCES OF UNHEALTHY FATS

Saturated Fats: whole and 2% milk, butter, and cheese; lard, fatty cuts of meat, and tropical oils (palm, palm kernel, and coconut oil), cocoa butter.

Trans Fats: Any food or food product that contains the words "hydrogenated" or "partially hydrogenated" in the ingredients, vegetable shortenings, some margarine, processed food (e.g., crackers, snack foods, cookies), and fried foods.

Smart Choices Eating Guidelines

Choose Complex Carbohydrates and Green Vegetables

Carbohydrates provide the energy you need both to work out and to get through your day. Composed of fibers, starches, and sugars, they fall into two basic categories: complex carbohydrates and simple carbohydrates. Complex carbohydrates are good for you and are composed of fiber and starches. Unrefined whole grains, starchy vegetables, and legumes are examples of complex carbohydrates.

Simple carbohydrates include fruit, milk and milk products, vegetables, and sweeteners. We'll talk about those in the next section of this chapter.

Complex carbohydrates are the right carbohydrates for weight loss because they are digested slowly, thus leaving you satisfied and providing you with steady energy. Foods made with unrefined or whole grains maintain their nutrients and contain important vitamins, minerals, and fiber, which help you avoid food cravings. Fiber adds bulk to your food, thereby contributing to your feeling of fullness. Fiber does not cost you a calorie because it cannot be digested.

The best way to determine if a product is made from whole grain is to read the label. According to a Mayo Clinic report on whole grains, "Many foods made from whole grains come ready to eat. These include a variety of breads, pasta products, and ready-to-eat cereals."[9] Whole grains should appear among the first few items in the ingredient list.

There is confusion about products made with flour. Whole-grain flour is made by grinding the entire grain, including the bran and the germ. Thus nutrients and fiber remain intact. If the bran and germ are removed during the milling process, the once whole grain is now dubbed a refined grain. You don't want to eat a blend of whole-grain and refined grain. You want only whole-grain in your food.

When you read the label and see whole-wheat specified, don't stop reading! Check to see if a refined grain is also listed, such as "enriched wheat flour" or "unbleached wheat flour." If it is then you are dealing with a blended product.

Do not be fooled by industry-generated marketing terms such as "made with," "good source of," "excellent source of," "multigrain," "100 percent wheat," and "contains whole grain" to name a few. These phrases allow manufacturers to blend their products with refined grains. If it does not say "100 percent whole grain" or "100 percent whole wheat," it's not for you!

Whole Grains	Refined Grains
Oatmeal	Enriched macaroni or pasta
Brown rice, wild rice	Pretzels
Whole-wheat bread, pasta, crackers	White bread
Barley, buckwheat, bulgur, millet	White rice
Popcorn	Corn flakes
	Couscous
	Grits

Smart Choices Eating Guidelines

Complex carbohydrates help you avoid food cravings because they enter the bloodstream at a slower rate than simple carbohydrates, thus raising blood sugar levels gradually. Whenever you eat carbs of any kind your body releases insulin in response. Insulin both helps your cells to absorb the energy you need and clears excess sugar from your bloodstream. If the insulin clears the excess sugar too quickly, causing blood sugar to plummet, the brain gets the message that you desperately need to eat. A slower digestion process enables your blood sugar levels to remain more stable, which tells your brain that you've satisfied your hunger.

You can never go wrong with green vegetables, such as broccoli, asparagus, brussels sprouts, green beans, zucchini, spinach, and my all-time favorite, romaine lettuce. The good news is you can eat all the green veggies you want because they contain so few carbs, and the carbs that they do contain are packed with fiber, causing them to be digested slowly. Non-green veggies, such as carrots, corn, and tomatoes have a higher sugar content and therefore should be eaten in limited quantities, as you want to stick to the guideline of eating low- to no-sugar foods.

A good rule of thumb is to add a splash of color to your primary green vegetable repertoire. Dice up a palm-sized portion of red peppers, onions, and carrots to sauté (with the help of a nonstick spray). Either toss this in with your green vegetable dish, or put it on the side. You can even use it as a garnish for your protein selection.

> **Complex Carbohydrates:** Whole grains (brown rice, whole-wheat bread, oatmeal, whole-wheat pasta, whole-grain cereal, wild rice), legumes, sweet potatoes.
>
> **Vegetables:** Broccoli, asparagus, brussels sprouts, green beans, zucchini, spinach, cabbage, romaine lettuce, among others.
>
> **Fruit:** Strawberries, blueberries, apples, pears, and others.

Fruit Is Good for You . . . in Moderation

When you eat fruit, stick to real, natural whole fruits. Although they have sugar, they are not stripped of fiber. Fiber enables fruit to be digested gradually, without causing blood sugar to spike. Fruit juice is not a good substitute for whole fruit because it lacks fiber and often contains added sugar. And beware: some fruits, such as bananas and grapes, are higher in sugar than others, so reach for strawberries, blueberries, and apples instead.

Be mindful. As you are striving for your first weight loss goal, you may want to stay away from fruit as it contains natural simple sugar and may affect the stability of your blood sugar and trigger hunger pangs. Although a little fruit in the morning may keep your sugar cravings in check, if you are anything like me, chances are you'll be left wanting more. In order to jump-start your results, avoid fruit for two or three weeks. Once you reach one or two of your goals you can reintroduce fruit.

Smart Choices Eating Guidelines

Even now, I tend to eat fruit in the morning before lunch. If you just can't imagine not eating fruit, eat one piece a day or half a cup of fruit slices or berries spread over your first two meals of the day, perhaps in a shake.

THE LOWDOWN ON THE GLYCEMIC LOAD

Perhaps you've heard of the glycemic index (GI), which ranks individual carbohydrates by how quickly they elevate blood glucose levels: classifying them as high, medium, and low. A measured portion of the food containing 50 g of available carbohydrates is necessary to determine the glycemic index of a food. Low GI carbohydrates tend to be the smartest choices because they produce only gradual variations in blood sugar. But—and it's a big but—a host of factors can lower or raise the GI of a food.

First, consuming protein and fat along with a carb slows digestion, leading to a more gradual rise in blood sugar levels than eating the carb alone. Second, the riper a fruit is the higher its GI will be. Third, longer cooking times soften food thereby making it easier to digest. This leads to a higher GI.

The concept of Glycemic Load (GL) is another useful tool for comparing individual carbs. It is more accurate than GI since it compares food by typical portion sizes rather than by weight. We don't eat all foods in the same portions, right? This means that carrots, for example, which are high GI, are low GL as most people only eat about a half a cup of carrots at a time.

Another example is watermelon. Watermelon comes in with a high GI ranking, but it would take four and a half cups of watermelon to match the GI standard measure (fifty grams). GL is applicable to everyday eating practices. When the GL of watermelon is calculated using a typical serving size of one-half cup, the GL is very low and allowable.

Like the Glycemic Index, the ranking system for the Glycemic Load is divided into three categories, namely low GL (ten or less), medium GL (eleven to nineteen), and high GL (twenty and above). It is an excellent guide for weight loss.

For more information on the Glycemic Index and Glycemic Load and to find the actual ratings of different foods visit: www.glycemicindex.com.

Beware of Simple and Refined Carbohydrates

Other than fruit, milk, milk products, and vegetables, most simple carbohydrates do not contain much in the way of nutritional value. Simple carbohydrates are found in sweeteners, such as refined sugar, honey, and corn syrup, and foods made with refined flour, such as bread. Foods made with simple refined carbohydrates are the wrong carbs for weight loss because they get absorbed into the blood stream quickly, thus raising blood sugar levels, which first creates a surge of energy and then a low, leaving you unsatisfied and craving a pick-me-up.

If you try to satisfy hunger pangs with more refined foods or simple carbohydrates, you will perpetuate a cycle of hunger and overeating. There is also a greater chance that the food you eat will be converted into fat and stored in your body.

Refined sugars provide empty calories because they lack vitamins, minerals, and fiber and therefore can lead to weight gain.

SOURCES OF UNHEALTHY CARBOHYDRATES[11]

Sweeteners: Refined sugar, honey, and corn syrup

Refined Flour Products (See "The Scoop on Grains" on page 29)

Smart Choices Eating Guidelines

Choose Healthy Protein

Protein is the main building block of muscles, organs, and glands. Every living cell and all body fluids, with the exception of bile and urine, contain protein. Protein in your diet plays an important role because it provides amino acids that the human body requires for the synthesis of its proteins. The body can make only thirteen of the amino acids necessary for the synthesis of its proteins. These are known as nonessential amino acids. The other nine essential amino acids can only be obtained from food.[12] Protein in your diet feeds and maintains your muscles and helps your body repair cells and make new ones.

Healthy protein comes from low-fat and high-fiber sources. Lean cuts of meat are a great source of protein as are legumes and egg whites. Other good sources of protein are powders, such as pure whey protein and high-protein, low-carb meal-replacement shakes. Vegetarians will obtain most of their protein from combination proteins found in foods such as brown rice and black beans or lentils. Protein shakes will come in handy for vegetarians in their quest to take in the appropriate amount of protein for their specific goals.

Note: The subject of complete and incomplete proteins is too big for this book. If you are a vegetarian, seek more information on the subject of vegetarian nutrition from a good reference guide, such as www.vrg.org.

To maintain rather than burn muscle during your workouts, you must eat enough protein. A common rule of thumb among the sports nutrition community is to consume one gram of protein per pound of your desired weight. This way you'll fuel your activities by burning your stored fat and recently eaten carbohydrates.

This may sound like a lot of protein to eat over the course of a day, but thanks to the assistance of protein shakes, you can easily and deliciously meet your protein needs. According to Sheah Rarback, whom I met with in consultation for this book, protein shakes are a great way to contribute to the fulfillment of your protein requirements.

SOURCES OF GOOD PROTEIN[13]

Lean Meat: Lean meat (for example, ground hamburger containing no more than 4 percent fat), poultry (skinless chicken breast and ground turkey containing 7 percent or less fat), and fish (tilapia, mahi mahi, and salmon)

Legumes: Beans (black beans, edamame or soy beans, red kidney beans), peas (black-eyed peas, chickpeas), and lentils

Other: Egg whites, whey protein powder, ready-to-drink protein shakes, low-carb meal replacement shakes

Water and Other Fluids

You must hydrate, hydrate, and hydrate. The best source of fluid is water. Consume a minimum of eight to ten 8-ounce glasses a day and even more when exercising. Don't wait until you are thirsty to drink because by then it is too late. A good trick is to go grab a drink of water every time you finish going to the bathroom. That way every time you "empty," you are reminded to refill! It's a foolproof (or should I say full-bladder) process.

You've all heard this advice before. I was never able to abide by this rule until I understood that if my body did not get the water it needed, it would hold on to the little I drank in fear of dehydration, causing me to ... you guessed it, *bloat!*

So, never be without water handy. I prefer carrying the twenty-four-ounce sports bottles, one of which I go through at the gym first thing in the morning. That's three of my eight-ounce glasses of water right there.

Smart Choices Eating Guidelines

The rest of the day I live off five-calorie, sugar-free drink mixes because they really satisfy my sweet cravings. Add the flavor of your choice right into a gallon jug and throw it in the fridge. This is easier than having to repeatedly clean smaller pitchers.

If you drink soda, it should be diet soda, free of caffeine and clear. While diet soda is void of sugar and calories, most diet sodas contain other suspect ingredients such as caffeine and the chemical additive phosphoric acid, which contain no nutritional value and can be damaging in the long run. Caffeine, for instance, is highly addictive and can cause a host of side effects once the initial buzz wears off, such as headaches and anxiety. It is also a diuretic and therefore does nothing to keep your body hydrated. Phosphoric acid, on the other hand, can throw off the pH balance of the body, thus causing the body to release calcium from teeth and bones in an effort to stabilize its pH. The calcium is lost in the process. That being said, indulging in a diet soda is a smarter choice than eating a piece of chocolate cake, but if you can do without diet soda until your cheat day, it's better. Otherwise, try to limit your consumption to one a day. Always keep your goals in mind when making your choices.

Only drink beverages with caffeine in moderation—whether that means soda, tea, or coffee. But go ahead and have a cup of decaffeinated coffee or tea.

Daily Multivitamin

Take one—it's good for you. It's important to cover all your bases nutritionally. If you're breastfeeding, check with your doctor to see how long you should continue taking prenatal vitamins before switching to another kind of multivitamin.

Dessert

Now let's talk about dessert. Believe me, you can search the freezer section for a healthy ice cream or frozen yogurt, but you won't find one. I know because I've looked. You will not find one that meets our food guidelines. One may be low in carbohydrates but high in sugar. Another may be made with a sugar substitute, but it is high in carbohydrates—not to mention the calorie content.

So ladies, Jell-O Sugar Free Low Calorie Gelatin Snacks consisting of ten calories, zero fat, and zero sugar are your new best friends. Squirt a dollop of fat free whipped cream on one and have yourself a party!

Your Cheat Meal

Once a week, you get to cheat on the plan. Here are the rules for cheating. They are simple.

RULE #1:

Have a plan. Look at your calendar for the week and decide in advance how you want to spend your cheat meal. Do you want to cheat on Friday night out with the girls for dinner? Or do you want to save your cheat for Saturday-night takeout with your hubby?

Having a plan helps you stay on track!

RULE #2:

Maintain clean eating for your four other meals on the day of your planned cheat.

Smart Choices Eating Guidelines

RULE #3:

There is no rule for what you choose to eat as your cheat. Have a glass or two of wine, lather some warm, refined bread with honey butter, and sink you teeth into the entrée and dessert of your choice.

RULE #4:

Don't overeat or binge because your body will pay for this behavior later. Remember, you will have the opportunity to cheat again.

RULE #5:

Give yourself permission to enjoy your cheat. Think of it from this perspective: there are seven days in a week during which you eat five meals a day. That works out to thirty-five meals a week, only one of which you are indulging yourself. So *enjoy* it!

I find adhering to the discipline of the Smart Choices Eating Guidelines is easiest Monday through Friday, and I suspect you will too. You and your children probably have a routine of play dates, mommy and me activities, or—if you are lucky—preschool! If you did not have a routine before you started this program, your new lifestyle will give you structure, predictability, and discipline.

Although I view taking care of my body and fueling it properly as my job, it's harder to stay on track on Saturdays and Sundays than on weekdays because my husband and kids are home. Also, dinner guests or meals out with friends can throw off my routine. You can see why you need a game plan for your cheat meal to mentally prepare for the weekend temptations and unpredictability. So choose your cheat meal wisely.

I like to indulge in my cheat meal on a fun night: Friday. My son is excited that school is over, everyone is looking forward to the weekend, and

I know I have an excruciating SPIN® class the following morning to burn through the extra calories.

When you indulge yourself after eating clean consistently throughout the week, you are actually shocking your body. Allowing your body to take in a high number of "forbidden" calories at one sitting actually jumpstarts your metabolism into high gear because your body has to work harder to burn off the ingested calories. Once you resume your normal clean eating regimen after your planned indulgence, both you and your body will be more than pleased to get back on track.

As you progress and achieve more of your goals, you can play with the cheat meal concept a little by adding a second cheat, but do this only if you gauge that it won't adversely affect the goals that you've set for your body.

It is crucial to stay on course until your designated cheat meal. You may think it is safe to pop one little Hershey's Kiss into your mouth, but it may be a mistake. It is like a gateway drug: once you do it, your body will crave more of the same. That one Kiss can stimulate your appetite and tempt your sugar tooth to just one more, then another, and another. Before long, you say to yourself, "What the heck? I've already messed up," causing you to continue down the wrong path, leading to guilty depression and more poor choices.

It will all be worth it once you see the results. And it will become easier because you will like what you see! Most importantly, you must believe in yourself and your commitment to the process.

You determine your success. So you have to be mentally ready or you will not achieve your goals.

You are now equipped to make smart choices, whether you are eating at home or going out with friends. As you see the results, it will be easier because you will start to believe in it.

Smart Choices Eating Guidelines

Condiments, Seasonings, Spices, and Sweeteners

The same basic principle of eating clean applies to flavor enhancers. Think salt free, sugar free, low carb, and low fat. I have included a list of my favorite brands at the back of the book (see page 135). And for you worrywarts, according to the National Cancer Institute, there is no evidence to support that there is an association between the use of artificial sweeteners and cancer.[14]

When and How to Eat Your Meals

Now that you know the right types of food to eat, let's discuss when and how to eat them. As moms of young children, we all lack time. There aren't enough hours in a day to do everything that we need and want to get done. But following Smart Choices Eating Guidelines requires minimal time and effort: your choices are defined for you, and they're not technical.

More important, you won't feel deprived because you're going to eat at least five small meals a day. That's right ladies, count them … I said *five!* At times it may feel like you are forcing yourself to eat when you start this regimen.

A key to the Smart Choices Eating Guidelines is to divide your caloric requirements among your meals. You should eat your calories in equal proportion: one-fifth per meal—give or take a few calories—or one-fourth of the calories for three main meals and one-eighth of your calories for two snacks. Or find the balance that works for you. I typically eat a similar amount of calories for my breakfast and my first snack of the day and then have slightly more calories for lunch. My second snack of the day usually is approximately half the calories of my first snack; I eat it just for a pick-me-up to keep my metabolism going. Then I balance the calories out at dinner.

It is important that you find a way of dividing the calories that makes sense for you. The point is not to overeat but to keep your metabolism going. Pay attention to the signals your body gives you and eat accordingly.

If you find that you've reached a plateau (meaning your weight change has become stagnant), you could cut your snack calories in half. This dilemma may indicate that it's time to reassess your caloric requirements, especially if you have made progress toward your goal.

The point of the eating guidelines is to help you make smart, informed choices. As with everything else in life, it takes time to acquire the knowledge that will empower you to succeed. It is important to remember that the long-term goal is good health and fitness not counting calories.

Eventually the eating guidelines will become second nature and you will be able to make your smart choices without blinking an eye or counting a calorie!

If you haven't already determined your total caloric requirement, go back to the formula in Chapter 2, page 17, and do it now.

When you eat less than your necessary caloric intake, your body will begin holding on to some of the calories you have eaten, storing them as fat in fear of starvation rather than processing them appropriately. A healthy metabolism burns through them on the spot. Eating exactly the amount of calories your body needs and can utilize at one time prevents it from storing anything as fat. And your body actually burns calories as it digests food! So how can you lose, or should I say not lose?

After a couple of weeks following the Eating Guidelines, you'll know exactly what a meal should feel like and look like. In the next chapter, "Sample Menu Items," I'll give you examples.

The nutritional key to the Smart Choices Eating Guidelines is to eat protein, carbohydrates, and fat with every meal. You should eat the majority of your carbohydrate calories at the beginning of the day—up to and including lunchtime—and less for your second snack and your third meal of the day (dinner). Eat grains, rice, oatmeal, bread, fruits, and sweet or starchy vegetables early in the day.

Smart Choices Eating Guidelines

During dinner your carbohydrates will only come from the occasional legume and what color veggies, ladies? That's right, *green* veggies! Because the calories are minimal in green veggies, you can eat as many as you want.

You will consume the right amount of fat simply by following the eating guidelines. Consuming the appropriate serving sizes of lean protein, fruits such as avocadoes, nuts, cooking oils, and products that contain healthy carbs will automatically provide you with the fat you need.

Play the Comparative Nutrition Game

We're going to play a game because it is necessary to learn how to navigate through the nutrition labels on products in the supermarket in order to make smart choices. For many of you, the game will be like seeing the labels for the first time. If you currently view them the way I used to, you are only paying attention to the fat grams. That explains why I could never get my belly the way I wanted it—and that was before kids. Face it, knowledge is power. Let's play three rounds.

ROUND #1:

In the first round, compare two different nutrition fact labels for two different brands of oatmeal. The question is: Which is a smarter choice? The main components that you need to pay close attention to are serving size, calories, total fat, carbohydrates, sodium, and sugar.

To evaluate carbohydrates use this formula: total carbohydrates minus dietary fiber equals net impact carbohydrates (TC − DF = NIC). You can use this formula to calculate the number of carbs that count in almost any given product.

Here are the two product labels.

Nutrition Facts		
Serving Size 1 packet (28g)		
Servings Per Container 12		
Amount Per Serving		
Calories 100	Calories From Fat20	
		% Daily Value
Total Fat 2g		3%
Saturated Fat 0g		0%
Trans Fat 0g		
Cholesterol 0mg		0%
Sodium 80mg		4%
Total Carbohydrates 19g		6%
Dietary Fiber 3g		12%
Sugars 0g		
Protein 4g		

Nutrition Facts		
Serving Size 1 packet (43g)		
Servings Per Container About 20		
Amount Per Serving		
Calories 160	Calories From Fat20	
		% Daily Value
Total Fat 2g		3%
Saturated Fat 0g		0%
Trans Fat 0g		
Cholesterol 0mg		0%
Sodium 270mg		11%
Total Carbohydrates 33g		11%
Dietary Fiber 3g		12%
Sugars 13g		
Protein 4g		

Did you notice the difference between these two brands of oatmeal? Although they both have 2 grams of fat per serving, the one on the right has 15 more grams per serving, 60 more calories, and 190 more mg of sodium. Using the Net Impact Formula, we can determine that the oatmeal on the right has 30 *carbs that count* (TC 33 – DF 3 = 30 NIC). It also contains 13 grams of sugar.

The oatmeal on the left by comparison has 16 carbs that count (TC 19 – DF 3 = 16 NIC) and 0 grams of sugar. In this instance, the oatmeal on the right just happens to be flavored while the oatmeal on the left is plain, which is a bit of a qualitative drawback. But you tell me, which is a smarter choice for weight loss? Correct: the one on the left.

Remember, the key to this lifestyle is controlling your carbohydrates and protein at every meal and eating low sodium and no to low sugar. Following these parameters will help you to make the right choices.

Smart Choices Eating Guidelines

ROUND #2:

In the second round, compare nutrition fact sheets for two different brands of whole-wheat bread. You've already checked the ingredient list and know that neither has refined flour in it. Which is the smarter choice, the label on the right or the left?

Nutrition Facts		
Serving Size 1 slice (26g)		
Servings Per Container 22		
Amount Per Serving		
Calories 50	Calories From Fat 10	
		% Daily Value
Total Fat 1g		1%
Saturated Fat 0g		0%
Trans Fat 0g		
Cholesterol 0mg		0%
Sodium 115mg		5%
Total Carbohydrates 10g		3%
Dietary Fiber 2g		8%
Sugars 1g		
Protein 4g		

Nutrition Facts		
Serving Size 1 slice (38g)		
Servings Per Container About 18		
Amount Per Serving		
Calories 100	Calories From Fat 10	
		% Daily Value
Total Fat 1g		2%
Saturated Fat 0g		0%
Trans Fat 0g		
Cholesterol 0mg		0%
Sodium 190mg		8%
Total Carbohydrates 30g		6%
Dietary Fiber 3g		12%
Sugars 6g		
Protein 4g		

It is easy to note significant differences right away among the main components of these breads. Although both breads contain 1 gram of fat per serving, the bread on the right has 12 more grams, 50 more calories, and 75 more milligrams of sodium per serving than the bread on the left. Using our handy-dandy NIC formula, we discover that the bread on the right has 27 carbs that count (TC 30 – DF 3 = 15 NIC) and 6 grams of sugar, while the bread on the left has 8 carbs that count (TC 10 – DF 2 = 8 NIC) and only 1 gram of sugar.

Now you tell me, which is the smarter choice? Correct: the one on the left.

ROUND #3:

In this final round of our game, we'll compare nutrition fact labels for two different brands of protein bars. Although these two protein bars start out looking similar in terms of serving size, calories, and fat grams, their differences become more apparent in the remaining components. But there's a new wrinkle in this more advanced round of our game; we're going to add a new factor to the formula for determining carbs that count.

Net impact carbs only include carbs that elevate your blood sugar level. If a type of carb cannot be digested and absorbed, such as fiber, it is deemed "unavailable." Therefore you can subtract these carbs from total carbs. In addition to dietary fiber, carbs falling into this category include sugar alcohols, glycerin, and glycerol. You'll find that this advanced information matters most when you're looking at low-calorie products that emulate sweets and candy, such as protein bars and chewing gum.

For your reference, some of the most common sugar alcohols are sorbitol, mannitol, maltitol, erythritol, and hydrogenated starch hydrolysates. Other sugar alcohols include xylitol, isomalt, and lactitol. What a mouthful!

Let's get back to our game. Notice that the protein bar labels below do not list glycerin, although they use it as an ingredient. The protein bar on the right excludes sugar alcohols on its label because they are not ingredients, which explain its higher sugar count of thirteen grams. However, the protein bar on the left notes on its packaging that the sugar alcohol count combined with the glycerin count equals fourteen grams.

Now you tell me, which is the smarter choice?

Smart Choices Eating Guidelines

Nutrition Facts		
Serving Size 1 bar (50g)		
Amount Per Serving		
Calories 190	Calories From Fat 50	
		% Daily Value
Total Fat 6g		9%
Saturated Fat 3g		15%
Trans Fat 0g		
Cholesterol 10mg		3%
Sodium 230mg		5%
Total Carbohydrates 17g		6%
Dietary Fiber 1g		4%
Sugars 2g		
Sugar Alcohol 7g		
Protein 20g		

Nutrition Facts		
Serving Size 1 bar (50g)		
Amount Per Serving		
Calories 210	Calories From Fat 60	
		% Daily Value
Total Fat 7g		11%
Saturated Fat 4g		20%
Trans Fat 0g		
Cholesterol <5mg		<2%
Sodium 330mg		14%
Total Carbohydrates 21g		7%
Dietary Fiber <1g		<4%
Sugars 13g		
Protein 16g		

The protein bar on the right has sodium content 100 milligrams higher than the protein bar on the left. It has 20 carbs that count (TC 21 – DF <1 = 20 NIC) and 13 grams of sugar.

By contrast, the protein bar on the left has 2 carbs that count (TC 17 – DF 1 – SA & G 14 = 2 NIC) and 2 grams of sugar. This bar would be my choice.

I prefer to buy products that spell out the net impact carb count or provide me enough detailed information to make an informed decision.

Love Your Smart Choices

As your palate adjusts to the allowable foods and you become more accustomed to making smart choices, I promise that your creativity will kick in and you'll learn to make simple meals more enticing. Congratulations! You are now eating to live not living to eat. This fact may make the initial adjustment easier. You will learn to love the smart choices you make because they'll boost your energy, trim your waistline, and help you accomplish your goals. You are sure to love the results.

In the next chapter, you'll find ready-made menu options to make your life easier.

Smart Choices Eating Guidelines

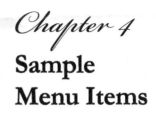

Chapter 4

Sample
Menu Items

*N*ow that we have established your food guidelines, let's put them to practical use. The parameters of our menu provide for three main meals (breakfast, lunch, and dinner) and two snacks (one midmorning and one midafternoon). Therefore, you'll be eating five small meals a day, approximately two and a half to three hours apart. Adhering to this schedule increases metabolism, reduces cravings, lowers body fat, and maintains energy levels.

Sound good? I thought so! What's on the menu?

Breakfast: Main Meal #1

In the beginning, keep your breakfasts simple. Once you get used to your new way of eating and feel more comfortable about combining the nutritional components of the Smart Choices Eating Guidelines, you can be more creative.

Here is how I think about breakfast: What will be my source of protein and what will be my source of carbohydrates? You need to have protein at every meal of the day to maintain muscle. You need to have carbs early in the day to give you energy for your activities. You'll taper off the carbs later in the day.

A Quick Note about Protein: On most days, you will be consuming a Whey Protein Shake as part of your breakfast unless your protein selection for this meal is combined with your carbohydrate selection as in the recipes for Protein Pancakes and the Protein Infusion Shake. Whey protein is a high quality protein powder derived from cow's milk during the cheese making process. It is a perfect source of protein.

I have compiled a list of simple breakfast choices for you to pull from when constructing your meal plan.

Breakfast Options

Oatmeal	Whole-Wheat Toast	Whole-Grain Cereal	Eggwich Delight	Friendly French Toast	Protein Pancakes	Protein Infusion Shake

IN A RUSH? "WHEY" YOUR OPTIONS

On those inevitable frantic mornings, finding the time to concoct even the simplest breakfast may seem impossible. Don't fret, here comes whey to the rescue!

Rather than blending your whey protein powder with ice and water, simply add one scoop of your powdered whey directly into your cooked oatmeal or dry cereal (it is easier to mix your whey powder into your cereal before you add your soymilk).

It is good to have a couple of different flavors of powder in the house for those mornings you are in a rush. For instance, I prefer vanilla-flavored whey in oatmeal but chocolate-flavored whey in cereal. Whey powder comes in a sufficient variety of flavors to satisfy everyone. Not only is the powdered version of whey protein easier on your budget, but it also goes a long way.

Ready-to-drink protein shakes are usually a blend of whey protein and soy protein. They are a fast on-the-go option but prepare to pay top dollar for them. Do your research to find the best buy.

Sample Menu Items

Whey Protein Shake

Whey Protein Shakes are a part of all the breakfast meals I recommend. After you experiment for a while you will learn exactly how you like your shake: creamier or icier, more water with less ice or lots of ice and lots of water. It is definitely a matter of personal taste.

Ingredients

1 scoop of whey protein powder

1 cup of water (more if desired)

Ice as desired

Instructions

Blend whey protein powder, water, and ice.

*Optional: Substitute whey protein shake with a ready-to-drink version (no preparation required).

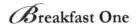

Oatmeal with Blueberries and a Whey Protein Shake

Nothing could be simpler than this quick-fix meal that fills you up and gives you the energy you need to start your morning.

Ingredients

1 packet of plain instant oatmeal

2/3 cup water

1 packet of sugar substitute (optional)

A handful, no more than a 1/4 cup of blueberries or another fruit such as strawberries (optional)

1 scoop whey protein powder (optional)

Instructions

Mix oatmeal and water in a microwave-safe cup or bowl. "Nuke" for one minute.

*Optional: Stir sugar substitute or mix berries into the cooked oatmeal or do both. Mix whey protein powder into oatmeal or drink as a shake (see recipe on page 52). Substitute a ready-to-drink protein shake for the Whey Protein Shake.

Breakfast One contains approximately 230 calories, 3.5 grams fat, 20 grams carbs, 1 gram sugar, and 28 grams protein.

Note: All calories listed in this chapter are for meals without the optional items. Feel free to alter the portion size based on your unique caloric requirements.

Sample Menu Items

Whole-wheat Toast with Green Apple Slices and a Whey Protein Shake

If you're a bread lover, this healthy breakfast combination will do the trick.

Ingredients

2 slices of whole-wheat bread, toasted

1/2 tablespoon sugar–free jelly per slice

A handful, no more than 1/4 cup of green apple slices or another fruit such as pear, served on the side (optional)

Whey Protein Shake (see recipe on page 52)

Instructions

Toast bread to your liking and spread with sugar-free jelly.

*Optional: Substitute a ready-to-drink protein shake for the Whey Protein Shake (no preparation required).

Breakfast Two contains approximately 230 calories, 4 grams fat, 26 grams carbs, 1 gram sugar, and 30 grams protein.

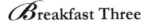

Whole-grain Cereal with Berries and a Whey Protein Shake

I gauge a cereal's carbohydrates by comparing them to my whole-wheat toast and oatmeal. I prefer a cereal that allows me a bigger serving size so that I don't have to eat less to stay in the appropriate carb range.

The serving size varies according to brand, so check the nutrition label. Most are good sources of carbs. You should be looking for a low carb to sugar ratio (and no more than two to three grams of sugar per serving). Use the Net Impact Carb formula in Chapter 3 on page 42, to calculate how many carbs you should be eating.

Ingredients

1 serving (may vary from 1/2 cup to 1-1/2 cups depending on brand) of cereal containing whole-grain ingredients, such as buckwheat, barley, oats, brown rice, or rye

4 ounces of plain light soymilk

1 packet of sugar substitute (optional)

A handful of berries (Example: blueberries, strawberries) no more than 1/4 cup (optional), mixed into the cereal, if desired

Whey Protein Shake (see recipe on page 52)

Instructions

Pour cereal and milk into bowl or to-go cup.

*Optional: Mix whey protein powder into cereal. If you do this, don't include the sugar substitute because the cereal will have plenty of flavor. You could also substitute a ready-to-drink protein shake for the Whey Protein Shake.

Breakfast Three contains approximately 260 calories, 3.25 grams fat, 26 grams carbs, 2 grams sugar, and 30 grams protein.

Sample Menu Items

Eggwich Delight with Cantaloupe and a Whey Protein Shake

Some people eat eggs every day for breakfast. If I had more time on my hands, I would eat them more often. Plan to eat them at least once a week.

Ingredients

1/4 to 1/2 cup egg substitute

Nonstick cooking spray

Seasoning to taste (see guidelines Chapter 3, page 40)

1 whole-wheat English Muffin, toasted

1 slice fat-free American cheese

A handful of cantaloupe pieces, no more than a 1/4 cup, or another fruit such as green apple, served on the side (optional)

Whey Protein Shake (see recipe on page 52)

Instructions

Pour the egg substitute onto a griddle sprayed with nonstick cooking spray and set to medium heat. Season as desired and scramble until the eggs reach the desired texture. Toast one whole-wheat English Muffin to your liking. To assemble, place the cooked scrambled eggs on one slice of the English Muffin, top with the slice of fat free American cheese, and cover with the remaining slice of English Muffin.

*Optional: Substitute a ready-to-drink protein shake, for the Whey Protein Shake.

Breakfast Four contains approximately 290 calories, 3.5 grams fat, 25 grams carbs, 2 grams sugar, and 41 grams protein.

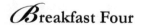

Try these variations:

Breakfast Omelet: Using the same base ingredients make an omelet and add the veggies of your choice and protein such as diced turkey slices to your egg substitute. You can even add a dash of fat-free cheese. Serve it with two slices of whole-wheat toast on the side, topped with sugar-free jelly or imitation butter spray. Don't forget your Whey Protein Shake and optional handful of fruit slices.

Breakfast Burritos: Feeling Southwestern? Add the veggies of your choice to your egg substitute and scramble to your liking. Place scrambled eggs into two whole-wheat tortillas and sprinkle with a dash of fat-free cheese and a tablespoon of fresh salsa. Don't forget your Whey Protein Shake and optional handful of fruit slices.

Sample Menu Items

Friendly French Toast with Berries and a Whey Protein Shake

This is a great treat to look forward to on a Sunday morning. Read the newspaper, have your husband take your kids for a walk, and eat your French toast in silence.

Ingredients

2 slices whole-wheat bread

1/4 cup egg substitute

1/8 cup plain soymilk

A dash of cinnamon

Imitation butter spray (optional)

1/4 cup Sugar-free, low-carb syrup (optional)

A handful of raspberries or blueberries, no more than 1/4 cup (optional)

Whey Protein Shake (see recipe on page 52)

Instructions

Mix egg substitute, soymilk, and cinnamon. Dip whole-wheat bread slices in the liquid mixture, coating both sides. Spray a griddle with nonstick cooking spray and set to medium-high heat. Cook both sides of the bread until golden brown. To serve, slice into triangular halves.

*Optional: Top with imitation butter spray and up to 1/4 cup of sugar-free, low-carb syrup. You may also garnish with a handful of berries, if desired. Substitute a ready-to-drink protein shake for the Whey Protein Shake.

Breakfast Five contains approximately 265 calories, 3.5 grams fat, 23 grams carbs, 1 gram sugar, and 36 grams protein.

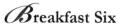

Protein Pancakes with Strawberries

This is a wonderfully filling breakfast if you're super hungry and want to pretend you're eating more than you actually are.

Ingredients

1 packet of plain oatmeal

1/2 cup of egg whites

1 scoop of whey protein powder (the flavor of your choice)

Nonstick cooking spray

1/4 cup sugar free, low-carb syrup (optional)

A handful (no more than ¼ cup) of strawberries or another fruit, sliced (optional)

Instructions

Combine oatmeal, egg whites, and whey protein powder to make a batter. Spray griddle with nonstick cooking spray. Pour a third of the batter onto a griddle set to medium-high heat. Flip the pancake when the edges begin to firm up, and the center of the pancake becomes porous. Makes approximately three good-sized pancakes.

*Optional: Spray with imitation butter spray and top with up to 1/4 cup sugar-free, low-carb syrup and/or garnish with a small handful of fruit.

Breakfast Six contains approximately 290 calories, 3.5 grams fat, 22 grams carbs, 1 gram sugar, and 40 grams protein.

Sample Menu Items

Protein-Infusion Shake

If you are feeling lazy or want a liquid breakfast, this is the solution.

Ingredients

1 packet of plain oatmeal

1 scoop of whey protein powder (the flavor of your choice)

1 cup of water (more if desired)

Ice, as desired

A handful of blueberries and/or strawberries (no more than 1/4 cup) or another fruit such as raspberries (optional)

Instructions

Blend oatmeal, whey protein powder, water, and ice.

*Optional: Put a handful of berries into the blender.

Breakfast Seven contains approximately 230 calories, 3.5 grams fat, 20 grams carbs, 1 gram sugar, and 28 grams protein.

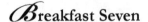

Breakfast Beverage Options

The consumption of a Whey Protein Shake might quench your thirst. However, if you are accustomed to drinking juice as a part of your morning ritual, you may initially find it difficult to forego that sweet sensation.

Don't worry! This is where a flavored, sugar-free drink mix with less than five calories comes in handy. Drink mixes like Crystal Light, 4C Totally Light, or a generic brand are a great way to satisfy your juice cravings while simultaneously contributing to your daily fluid intake. And let's not forget about good, old-fashioned water, which is always a great option.

One cup of coffee or tea in the morning won't hurt you. However, if you are consuming coffee out of habit or because you like the taste rather than for a caffeine boost, opt for caffeine-free coffee or tea instead.

Sample Menu Items

Midmorning Snack

If you exercise in the morning, be sure to consume this meal shortly after your intense workout so that your energy level stays high until lunch. Whether you have just completed thirty minutes of weight training, an hour of kick boxing, or pulled off a great PowerPoint presentation on four hours of sleep (thanks to your little angel), your midmorning snack serves the same function. It is a great way to fulfill your protein requirement, replenish your body's fuel, feed your muscles, and keep your metabolism chugging along.

Simplicity is the key to staying on the plan, and it doesn't get simpler than this. You have three options for your morning snack: a shake, a bar, and "real" food.

Another option is to swap out your midmorning snack for lunch, a.k.a. Main Meal Two. It might be easier to swing by your favorite wrap shop and save your shake for the next meal. Remember: there is always a way to make the right choice.

Midmorning Snack Options

High-protein, Low-carb Meal-Replacement Shake	Protein Bar	Real Food Option (1 carb/1 protein)

High-protein, Low-carb Meal-Replacement Shake

My personal choice, hands down, is a Lean Body for Her meal-replacement shake. It provides me with thirty grams of protein, and it is a perfect pick-me-up after my intense workout at the gym. These types of drinks are light, refreshing, and provide a perfectly balanced blend of nutrients. And yes ladies, there are a variety of flavors to choose from to satiate your particular craving.

You can add fruit to your shake once you reach a goal or two, but these shakes are so yummy it isn't necessary. They are super simple and super quick. Just add water, ice, and blend. You can even just add water and shake it vigorously in a thermos if you're really in a rush, which I've done on numerous occasions.

Ingredients

1 high-protein, low-carb meal-replacement shake packet

1 cup water (more if desired)

A handful of ice (more if desired)

A handful (no more than a 1/4 cup) of blueberries or another fruit such as strawberries (optional)

Instructions

Fill blender with water, ice, and the contents of the packet. Blend to desired consistency.

*Optional: You may add a handful of fruit directly into the blender, if desired. Or you can substitute a ready-to-drink, high-protein, meal-replacement shake (no preparation required).

(Midmorning Snack One continued on next page)

Sample Menu Items

If you're watching your pennies due to the expense of your new baby, you can use your whey protein to make your own meal-replacement shake (see recipe for Breakfast Seven, "Protein-Infusion Shake," on page 60)

Midmorning Snack One contains approximately 180 calories, 3 grams fat, 6 grams carbs, 1 gram sugar, and 30 grams protein.

THE PERFECT MEAL ... REPLACEMENT

A meal-replacement shake is just that ... a shake that replaces a meal. They are formulated to have a healthy balance of carbohydrates, protein, and fat as well as vitamins and minerals. They are typically low in sugar, yet with a little artificial sweetener they have just enough flavor to be enticing.

As with everything else, you must always read the nutrition labels before making a decision about what meal replacement shake is right for you. Make sure to choose one that has a ratio of protein, carbohydrates, fat, and sugar that aligns with your goals.

Protein Bar

The protein bar is great when you know you have to run a million errands after the gym and won't make it home in time to make a shake. My favorite protein bar is a Pure Protein bar. They come in a variety of flavors, so whether you are a fruit lover or a chocolate lover, Pure Protein has you covered.

Ingredients

1 protein bar

Instructions

Pack it, open it, and eat it! Oh yeah ... and enjoy it!

Midmorning Snack Two contains approximately 180 calories, 4.5 grams fat, 11 grams carbs, 2 grams sugar, and 20 grams protein.

Midmorning Snack Three

Real Food Option: Pick a Carb and Pick a Protein

If you have a hard time getting used to meal replacement shakes and/or protein bars, you can opt for a solid snack that consists of good, old-fashioned, regular food.

Ingredients

1/2 whole-wheat bagel or 1 mini bagel (toasted, if desired)

3-4 ounces of oven-roasted, low-sodium, sliced turkey breast

A handful of the veggies of your choice (romaine lettuce, alfalfa sprouts, one thin tomato slice, one thin onion slice)

Seasoning, to taste (see guidelines Chapter 3, page 40)

Imitation butter spray (optional)

1 tablespoon mustard (optional)

A handful (no more than 1/4 cup) of green apple slices or another fruit such as pear, served on the side (optional)

Instructions

If desired, toast your whole-wheat bagel or mini bagel halves to your liking. To assemble, place the turkey slices on the bagel and top with the veggies of your choice.

*Optional: Spray bagel with imitation butter spray or spread mustard onto bagel halves.

Midmorning Snack 3 contains approximately 210 calories, 2.75 grams fat, 15 grams carbs, 2.5 grams sugar, and 30.5 grams protein.

There is always a smart choice available to you. You could even prepare an Eggwich Delight or Protein Pancakes from the Breakfast Options if you're in the mood. (See recipe for Breakfast Option Four on page 56 and Breakfast Six on page 59).

Sample Menu Items

Lunch: Main Meal Two

This is your last daily opportunity to consume a healthy portion of the whole-grain carbohydrates that your body needs because after this meal you should taper off your carbs. Depending on your midafternoon snack choice, you may cut out carbs completely for the rest of the day. If you work out late in the day or early evening, however, you'll need the energy carbs provide to tide you over until dinner. If that is the case, make sure to choose one of the midafternoon snack choices that incorporate a form of carbohydrates, such as rice cakes.

If you are anything like me, you love eating carbs. That's okay! They are necessary and good for you, which is why—unlike some diets—the Smart Choices Eating Guidelines allow for their consumption. Just remember to practice portion control at every meal. Only consume what you need to burn during the next few hours.

When I think about building my lunch, three questions come to mind: Where will my protein come from? What complex carbohydrate will I choose? And, what will I do for a vegetable? I base my decision on what I'm in the mood for (a sandwich, a salad, pasta, a sweet potato?) and on what's leftover or available in the fridge. I tend to choose anything that will make my life easier.

Here are seven simple, smart choices!

Lunch Options

Lean Turkey Burger	Grilled Chicken Salad	Tuna Salad Pita	Grilled Tilapia	Pasta with Turkey Meatballs	Turkey Breast Sandwich	Protein Pancakes

> # *L*unch One

Lean Turkey Burger with Brown Rice and a Garden Salad

Welcome to the segment I like to call "101 Ways to Prepare Turkey." This is one of the easiest and tastiest ways to prepare it.

Ingredients

4 ounces of lean ground turkey molded into a patty. (Can substitute frozen turkey burger patty or veggie burger)

Seasoning, to taste (see guidelines Chapter 3, page 40)

1/2 cup instant brown rice (makes 2/3 cup cooked)

Imitation butter spray (optional)

1 cup romaine lettuce (more if desired)

A generous portion of your favorite veggies

2 tablespoons balsamic vinegar

Instructions

Frozen patty: follow the directions on the package. Fresh patty: season as desired. Broil or grill to your liking. Prepare 1/2 cup of instant brown rice as directed on package. Place half of the rice on your plate and reserve the other half for another day or, if your caloric requirements call for it, you may need to eat it now.

Prepare a side garden salad with romaine lettuce and the veggies of your choice such as cucumbers, grape tomatoes, green peppers, and so on. Top with balsamic vinegar. Serve on the side.

*Optional: You may spray your rice with an imitation butter spray.

Lunch One contains approximately 235 calories, 9.75 grams fat, 17 grams carbs, 0 grams sugar, and 23 grams protein.

Sample Menu Items

Grilled Chicken Salad on a Bed of Romaine Lettuce with a Baked Sweet Potato

Let me count the ways I love thee, Chicken … it is no wonder that I am growing feathers. You definitely can't beat this delicious yet nutritious lunch option.

Ingredients

4 ounces of boneless, skinless chicken breast

Imitation butter spray or 1/2 tablespoon olive oil

Seasoning, to taste (see guidelines Chapter 3, page 40)

1 cup of romaine lettuce (more if desired)

A generous portion of your favorite veggies

2 tablespoons balsamic vinegar

1 small sweet potato

1/8 cup almond slivers (optional)

Imitation butter spray (optional)

A dash of cinnamon (optional)

A sprinkle of sugar substitute (optional)

Instructions

Lightly coat chicken with imitation butter spray or olive oil. Grill or broil chicken breast. Slice cooked chicken to your liking and serve it on top of romaine lettuce. Add your favorite veggies and top with balsamic vinegar. Pierce sweet potato with a fork, and then cook it in the microwave for four minutes or until soft when tested with a fork.

(Lunch Two continued on next page)

*Optional: You may add a sprinkle (no more than 1/8 cup) of sliced almonds to your salad. You also may spray your sweet potato with an imitation butter spray and sprinkle it with a dash of cinnamon and sugar substitute.

Lunch Two contains approximately 186 calories, 0.17 grams fat, 15 grams carbs, 2.5 grams sugar, and 27 grams protein.

Sample Menu Items

Tuna Pita Salad

This is a great way to scale back your figure. You can never go wrong with tuna because it's packed full of protein.

Ingredients

3 ounces (1/2 can) of solid white albacore tuna, packed in water

1 tablespoon mustard (more if desired)

1/2 tablespoon low-fat mayonnaise (optional)

1 stalk celery, diced

1 medium onion slice diced

Seasoning, to taste (see guidelines Chapter 3, page 40)

1/2 whole-wheat low-carb pita bread pocket

1/2 cup shredded romaine lettuce

1/8 cup almond slivers (optional)

1 slice fat-free cheese (optional)

Favorite veggies (optional)

Instructions

Mix mustard and mayonnaise. Add a generous amount of diced celery and onion. Season as desired. Cut a whole-wheat pita in half (reserving the second half for another day) and scoop tuna salad into the pita pocket. Add shredded romaine lettuce to pita.

(Lunch Three continued on next page)

(Lunch Three continued from previous page)

*Optional: You may add a handful (no more than a 1/8 cup) of sliced almonds and/or a slice of fat-free cheese to your tuna salad pita. You may add the
veggies of your choice in addition to romaine lettuce.

Lunch Three contains approximately 235 calories, 5.5 grams fat, 7 grams carbs, 0
grams sugar, and 30.5 grams protein.

Sample Menu Items

Lunch Four

Grilled Tilapia with Brown Rice and Steamed Broccoli

If you dislike fishy tastes and smells, tilapia is a great fish choice for you. I enjoy fish that tastes like chicken (meaning nothing like fish) and have had great experiences with tilapia.

Ingredients

4 ounces of tilapia filet (or substitute mahi mahi)

Imitation butter spray (or 1/2 tablespoon olive oil)

2 tablespoons lemon juice

Seasoning, to taste (see guidelines, Chapter 3, page 40)

1/2 cup instant brown rice (makes 2/3 cup cooked), or substitute a sweet potato

1 cup broccoli florets (steamed)

Imitation Butter Spray (optional)

A dash of parmesan cheese (optional)

Instructions

Coat the tilapia filet with imitation butter spray or olive oil and squirt it with lemon juice. Season as desired. Grill or broil. Prepare 1/2 cup of instant brown rice as directed on package. Place half of the rice on your plate and reserve the other half for another day, or, if your caloric requirements call for it, you can eat it now. Or substitute a sweet potato for the rice (see Lunch Two, page 70, for details about preparation). Steam a hearty portion of broccoli in the microwave.

*Optional: You may spray your rice with imitation butter spray and season appropriately. You may spray your sweet potato with imitation butter and sprinkle with a dash of cinnamon and sugar substitute. You may spray your broccoli with imitation butter spray and add a dash of grated parmesan cheese.

(Lunch Four continued on next page)

(Lunch Four continued from previous page)

Lunch Four contains approximately 243 calories, 2 grams fat, 25 grams carbs, 1.5 grams sugar, and 33 grams protein.

Sample Menu Items

Turkey Meatballs on a Bed of Whole-Wheat Pasta with a Romaine Vegetable Salad

For all of you Italian carb lovers, this is amore.

Ingredients

2 ounces of whole-wheat pasta (dry), cooked and drained

4 ounces of lean ground turkey

1 clove of garlic, crushed

1/8 cup egg substitute

1 tablespoon parmesan cheese, grated

Salt-free garlic and herb seasoning

Salt-free Italian medley seasoning

Imitation butter spray (optional)

1/2 tablespoon olive oil (optional)

1/4 cup low-sugar, low-carb spaghetti sauce (optional)

A dash of parmesan cheese (optional)

1 cup romaine lettuce (more if desired)

A generous portion of your favorite veggies

2 tablespoons balsamic vinegar

Instructions

Combine ground turkey, crushed garlic, egg substitute, parmesan cheese, and seasonings. Shape mixture into two round meatballs. Broil in the oven until fully cooked (approximately twenty minutes), turning the meatballs once to brown

(Lunch Five continued on next page)

The Hot Mommy Next Door

(Lunch Five continued from previous page)

them evenly. Serve on top of pasta. Prepare a side salad of romaine lettuce and veggies, and top it with balsamic vinegar.

*Optional: You may spray your pasta with imitation butter, mix in 1/2 tablespoon of olive oil, or add 1/8 cup low-sugar, low-carb spaghetti sauce for taste. You may also add a dash of parmesan cheese.

Lunch Five contains approximately 375 calories, 9.75 grams fat, 35 grams carbs, 2 grams sugar, and 35 grams protein.

Sample Menu Items

Turkey Breast Sandwich with Steamed Asparagus

This dish is a classic example of eating what is available. You know you have turkey slices in the fridge, whole-wheat bread in the pantry, and steamed asparagus left over from last night's dinner. Decision made.

Ingredients

4 ounces of oven-roasted, low-sodium sliced turkey breast

Two pieces of whole-wheat bread (toasted, if desired)

1/2 tablespoon mustard

1/2 tablespoon low-fat mayonnaise (optional)

1/2 cup shredded romaine lettuce

Seasoning, to taste (see guidelines Chapter 3, page 40)

1 slice fat-free cheese (optional)

1 cup asparagus stalks, steamed

Favorite veggies (optional)

Instructions

Spread both slices of bread with mustard or one slice with 1/2 tablespoon low-fat mayonnaise and the other with mustard. Lay turkey slices inside and top with romaine lettuce. Serve with steamed asparagus on the side.

*Optional: In addition to the lettuce, you may add the veggies of your choice and a slice of fat-free cheese to your sandwich.

Lunch Six contains approximately 250 calories, 4 grams fat, 24 grams carbs, 2.5 grams sugar, and 35 grams protein.

Protein Pancakes

This breakfast item also makes a nice lunch (see recipe for Breakfast Six on page 59).

All seven of these lunch choices are quick and easy to prepare. And with the exception of the protein pancakes, whether you are craving a sandwich, salad, or pasta ... these lunches are interchangeable. For example, you could make a turkey meatball sandwich with a side salad rather than eating your meatballs over pasta. You could also opt to eat your turkey meatballs with a sweet potato and a side of broccoli, and so on.

To save time, you can cook extra protein the night before you'll need it. If you are grilling chicken breasts throw an extra on. If you are baking turkey burgers in the oven, toss another one in the pan. Then you'll only have to reheat it for lunch.

The same rule applies to your veggies: make extra. Then you'll only have to pop a sweet potato in the microwave for four minutes, cook a serving of five-minute brown rice, or pull out a bag of prepackaged lettuce, and you've got lunch.

Where would we moms be without today's modern conveniences? Quick and easy is my motto.

If you are lucky enough to time a midmorning nap for your little one so you can spend some "me" time socializing with friends at a restaurant, don't fret about your lunch options. No matter where you are, you can always make

Sample Menu Items

smart choices. The choices I've given you are easily adapted to the menus of most restaurants.

Remember: don't be afraid to speak up, ask questions, and make special requests of servers in order to take charge of your nutrition and calories while eating out.

Midafternoon Snack

You must keep eating throughout the day. It may feel difficult to snack in the beginning, especially if you've barely made time for two meals a day let alone five. But once your body gets used to its new eating habits, you will anticipate your next meal with a passionate (or at least hearty) hunger. Snacking keeps your blood sugar and metabolism constant. Remember, at this point in your day you are tapering off your carbs, so a protein-based snack is a good option. Some days that just won't cut it, however, so I have provided different options for different needs.

Again, the key is simplicity. So once more I have laid out some simple food choices for you.

Midafternoon Snack Options

Turkey Rolls	Canned Tuna	Rice Cakes w/PB&J	Yogurt Cup or Smoothie	Low-Fat Cottage Cheese	Whey Protein Shake	Protein Bar

Turkey Rolls with an Optional Brown Rice Cake

This is the way I roll.

Ingredients

3–4 ounces of oven roasted, low-sodium sliced turkey breast

1 brown rice cake, lightly salted (optional)

Mustard, to taste (optional)

Veggies of your choice (optional)

Instructions

Roll turkey slices and have at them.

*Optional: Smear a brown rice cake with mustard and lay turkey slices on top. Feel free to add veggies of your choice such as lettuce, onion, or alfalfa sprouts.

Snack One contains approximately 120 calories, 2 grams fat, 0 grams carbs, 0 grams sugar, and 26 grams protein.

Canned Tuna with an Optional Low-carb, Whole-wheat Wrap and Melted Cheese

How's this for a protein-packed, simple snack?

Ingredients

3 ounces (1/2 can) of solid white albacore tuna in water, plain or mixed with mustard

1 low-carb, whole-wheat wrap (optional)

1/8 cup fat-free cheese shredded (optional)

Instructions

Pop open the can of tuna and proceed to eat half.

*Optional: Mix tuna with desired amount of mustard. Or wrap it in one low-carb, whole-wheat tortilla with a sprinkle of shredded fat-free cheese microwave until the cheese is melted.

Snack Two contains approximately 105 calories, 3 grams fat, 0 grams carbs, 0 grams sugar, and 19.5 grams protein.

Rice Cakes with Peanut Butter and Jelly

Can you say, "Yummy in my tummy"? This was a staple snack for me during my weight loss journey. It's especially good if you do an afternoon workout because it provides a little more carbs than the other snacks.

Ingredients

2 lightly salted brown rice cakes

1 tablespoon or less low-sodium, reduced carbohydrate peanut butter

1 tablespoon sugar-free jelly

Instructions

Top each rice cake with a thin layer (no more than 1/2 tablespoon per rice cake) of peanut butter and 1/2 tablespoon of sugar-free jelly.

Snack Three contains approximately 175 calories, 8 grams fat, 21 grams carbs, 1 gram sugar, and 6 grams protein.

Sample Menu Items

Yogurt Cup or Yogurt Smoothie with Optional Raw Almonds

This is a great on-the-go snack option.

Ingredients

1 low-carb, low-sugar yogurt cup (4 ounces) or drinkable yogurt smoothie

8–10 raw almonds (optional)

Instructions

Remove the yogurt cup or yogurt smoothie from the fridge and eat or drink.

*Optional: Count out your almonds and eat them.

Snack Four contains approximately 60 calories, 3 grams fat, 3 grams carbs, 2 grams sugar, and 5 grams protein.

Low-fat Cottage Cheese
with Optional Celery Stalks and Peanut Butter

Say no to "cottage cheese" on your thighs by saying yes to cottage cheese as a snack.

Ingredients

1 4-ounce cup of low-fat cottage cheese

2 stalks of celery, cut in halves (optional)

1 tablespoon low-sodium, reduced carbohydrate peanut butter (optional)

A dash of cinnamon (optional)

1 tablespoon sugar-free jelly (optional)

Instructions

Remove cottage cheese cup from the fridge and eat.

Optional: Sprinkle cottage cheese cup with a dash of cinnamon or stir in a tablespoon of sugar-free jelly. Or spread the celery stalks with peanut butter and enjoy.

Snack Five contains approximately 90 calories, 2 grams fat, 5 grams carbs, 4 grams sugar, and 10 grams protein.

Sample Menu Items

Whey Protein Shake

This snack option is whey too easy! See recipe and caloric information for Whey Protein Shake, on page 52.

*Optional: Substitute a ready-to-drink protein shake for the Whey Protein Shake.

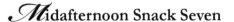

One-half Protein Bar

This is another quick fix for your nutritional needs. Simply cut a protein bar in half. Share the other half with a friend or save it for tomorrow's midafternoon snack. (See Midmorning Snack 2, page 65, for caloric information).

All seven midafternoon snack options are quick, simple, and easily transportable. Most of the time I eat this snack in the car on my way somewhere to drop off or pick up the kids. This meal provides me with the little boost of energy I need to survive until dinner—hours filled with playtime, bath time, dinnertime, and bedtime.

Dinner: Main Meal Three

It doesn't get any simpler than dinner, thank goodness. By the time you get to your fifth meal of the day (not to mention all the cooking you do for the kids) you probably don't want to think about food anymore. So here's your simple rule: Just pick a protein, pick a green veggie, and have at it.

Your protein serving can range anywhere from three to six ounces (depending on your caloric and protein requirements). Choose from lean meats and plant-based proteins like tofu. You can eat all the veggies you want from the food list in Chapter 3 (see page 31).

Please note, all the nutritional information in this section is based on a single portion size containing one cup of vegetables.

Dinner Options

Filet Mignon	Salmon Filet	Grilled Chicken	Turkey Burger	Take out	Pork Tenderloin	Omelet Surprise

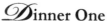
Filet Mignon with Onions and Mushrooms and Steamed Asparagus

I only treat myself to red meat once a week, so I like to find the top of the loin, I mean, line.

Ingredients

4 ounces of beef tenderloin, grilled to your liking.

2 medium onion slices, diced, (optional)

1/2 cup sliced mushrooms (optional)

1 tablespoon olive oil or nonstick cooking spray

Seasoning, to taste (see guidelines Chapter 3, page 40)

1 pound asparagus stalks

Imitation butter spray (optional)

A dash of parmesan cheese, grated (optional)

1/8 cup sliced almonds (optional)

Instructions

Season filet as desired and grill to your liking. Sauté diced onions and mushrooms in one tablespoon olive oil or nonfat cooking spray and then serve as a garnish or topping. Steam asparagus in the microwave for four to six minutes (save the leftovers for the next day).

*Optional: You may spray your asparagus with an imitation butter spray and season as desired. You may also top your asparagus with a dash of parmesan cheese and/or a sprinkle of sliced almonds.

(Dinner One continued on next page)

Sample Menu Items

Dinner One contains approximately 146 calories, 2.4 grams fat, 6 grams carbs, 2.5 grams sugar, and 27 grams protein.

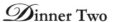
Salmon Filet with Steamed Broccoli

Salmon is a great dinner option. It's one of the so-called superfoods because it is so packed with nutrients.

Ingredients

4 ounces of salmon filet (or mahi mahi)

Imitation butter spray or 1/2 tablespoon olive oil

1 tablespoon lemon juice

1 pound broccoli florets

Seasoning, to taste (see guidelines Chapter 3, page 40)

Imitation butter spray (optional)

A dash of parmesan cheese, grated (optional)

Instructions

Spray Salmon with imitation butter or coat with 1 tablespoon olive oil and a squirt of lemon juice. Season as desired. Grill or bake according to your preference. Steam broccoli in the microwave for four to six minutes (and save the leftovers for the next day).

*Optional: You may spray your broccoli with imitation butter and add a dash of parmesan cheese.

Dinner Two contains approximately 205 calories, 8 grams fat, 8 grams carbs, 1.5 grams sugar, and 27 grams protein.

Sample Menu Items

Grilled Chicken with Steamed Brussels Sprouts

It's a good thing chicken is versatile and delicious because you will be eating a lot of it.

Ingredients

4 ounces of boneless, skinless chicken breast

Imitation butter spray

1 pound brussels sprouts

Seasoning, to taste (see guidelines Chapter 3, page 40)

A dash of parmesan cheese, grated (optional)

1/2 tablespoon olive oil (optional)

Instructions

Spray chicken breast with imitation butter spray. Season as desired. Grill or broil to your liking. Steam brussels sprouts until desired tenderness (save the leftovers for the next day).

*Optional: You may spray your Brussels sprouts with imitation butter or top with ½ tablespoon olive oil and season appropriately. You may also add a dash of parmesan cheese.

Dinner Three contains approximately 184 calories, 1 grams fat, 14 grams carbs, 2 grams sugar, and 30 grams protein.

Try these variations:

Grilled Chicken Salad: Make it a salad with romaine lettuce, cucumbers, sliced avocado, sliced almonds, and a handful of grape tomatoes. Don't forget the balsamic vinegar. Too tired to grill chicken? Pick up a rotisserie chicken, remove the skin, and chop up the chicken breast.

Friendly Fajitas: Line baking tray with foil and spray with nonstick cooking spray. Slice green peppers and onions, arrange them on baking tray, and spray them with nonstick cooking spray. Season to taste and broil them as desired. Line a separate baking tray with foil and spray with nonstick cooking spray. Arrange chicken breast tenderloins on baking tray, spray them with nonstick cooking spray, and season to taste. Broil on each side until cooked thoroughly and golden brown. Use two low-carb tortillas to make fajitas with chicken and vegetables. If desired, add a sprinkle of fat-free cheese, one tablespoon of fresh salsa, and a tablespoon of black beans.

Sample Menu Items

Turkey Burger with a Romaine Vegetable Salad

Can I get a gobble, gobble? Even my kids love these delicious burgers, so you know they must be tasty!

Ingredients

4 ounces of lean ground turkey molded into a patty.

Seasoning, to taste (see guidelines Chapter 3, page 40)

2 medium onion slices, diced (optional)

A dash of parmesan cheese, grated (optional)

1 slice fat-free cheese (optional)

Imitation butter spray (optional)

1 cup romaine lettuce (more if desired)

A generous portion of your favorite veggies

2 tablespoons balsamic vinegar

Instructions

Season burgers as desired. Grill or broil turkey burgers to your liking. Prepare a side salad of romaine lettuce and veggies, and top it with balsamic vinegar.

*Optional: You may mix diced onions, a dash of parmesan cheese, and seasoning directly into ground turkey before molding it into a patty. You may also add a slice of fat-free cheese. You may spray your asparagus with an imitation butter spray and season appropriately.

Dinner Four contains approximately 190 calories, 8 grams fat, 6 grams carbs, 2.5 grams sugar, and 26 grams protein.

Try this variation:

Turkey Chili: Four cloves of garlic crushed. Heat one tablespoon olive oil on medium-low heat and add garlic. Do not brown garlic. Next add one cup diced onions (color of your choice) and sauté with garlic until translucent. Add to the mix one pound of lean ground turkey and set cooktop to medium-high heat. Cook turkey thoroughly until it is brown.

You may choose to add some chili seasoning to the cooked ground meat, but use it sparingly (no more than one tablespoon) because it usually contains a lot of sodium. Next add one 14 1/2-ounce can of diced tomatoes (no sodium added) and one 16-ounce can of light red kidney beans (they typically have less sodium than dark red kidney beans) drained.

You can eat the turkey chili atop a bed of romaine lettuce in addition to your green vegetable of choice or just have it with a side of vegetables. You may add a sprinkle of fat-free cheese if desired. If you are in a carb frenzy that evening, you can make tacos by placing your serving of turkey chili into two low-carb, whole-wheat tortillas.

Sample Menu Items

Take Out

For when it has just been one of those days … instead of making dinner, make a phone call to your favorite Japanese restaurant. Order one Chicken Yakitori appetizer (grilled chicken and scallions on skewers) with no Teriyaki sauce, one order of Edamame (soy beans) with no salt, and a house salad with ginger dressing on the side (used sparingly or not at all). You could always grab your balsamic vinegar instead! I must have been Japanese in a past life because I eat this a lot!

*Optional: If you're extra hungry because you really kicked butt at the gym or if you have your period, you may want to sink your teeth into a carbohydrate that isn't green and leafy. Try ordering a California roll, which usually contains cucumber (a green veggie), avocado (a healthy fat source), and crab-meat protein wrapped in seaweed and brown rice. And it's a perfect portion size. Make sure to specify brown rice when ordering.

More than likely you will have some leftover chicken and probably half a roll, so you have lunch for the following day. But don't forget your green vegetable!

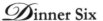
Pork Tenderloin with Steamed Green Beans

This is another simple dinner option that provides a nice break from the feather family.

Ingredients

4 ounces of lean boneless pork tenderloin

1 pound of green beans

Seasoning, to taste (see guidelines Chapter 3, page 40)

Imitation butter spray (optional)

1/8 cup sliced almonds (optional)

Instructions

Season pork tenderloin as desired. Grill or broil the tenderloin to your liking. Steam green beans in the microwave as directed on prepackaged bag (save the leftovers for lunch the next day).

*Optional: You may spray your green beans with an imitation butter spray and season appropriately. You may also add a sprinkle of sliced almonds.

Dinner Six contains approximately 169 calories, 5 grams fat, 10 grams carbs, 1.5 grams sugar, and 24 grams protein.

Sample Menu Items

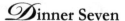

Dinner Seven

Omelet Surprise

I usually resort to this meal when Mama is just too tired to cook.

Ingredients

1/2 to 3/4 cup egg substitute (flavored, if you prefer)

1 cup vegetable medley, sautéed with nonstick cooking spray

3–4 ounces of oven-roasted, low-sodium, sliced turkey breast, diced

Nonstick cooking spray

Seasoning, to taste (see guidelines Chapter 3, page 40)

1/8 cup shredded fat-free cheese (optional)

1 tablespoon low-carb/low-sugar ketchup (optional)

Instructions

Pour the egg substitute onto a griddle sprayed with nonstick cooking spray and set to medium heat. Add previously sautéed vegetable medley and diced turkey breast. Season as desired and fold eggs over once the eggs are solid. (Some people prefer them moist; others prefer them dry. Cook them according to your taste.)

*Optional: You may add a dash of shredded fat-free cheese to your omelet. And the kid in you may want to dip your omelet sparingly into some low-carb and low-sugar ketchup.

Dinner Seven contains approximately 220 calories, 2 grams fat, 7 grams carbs, 3 grams sugar, and 39 grams protein.

Your Cheat Meal

A cheat meal could take the place of a breakfast, a lunch, or a dinner. Whenever you use this special meal, indulge and enjoy it. But remember not to binge! You've earned it, you've planned it, and you know that you will get to do it again next week. So don't try to fit everything you've been craving into one sitting. Book the indulgences you don't get this week for next week's cheat!

That is why we plan, ladies.

Your Cheat Meal should contain approximately ... oh, forget it. Who is counting calories? Delicious fat, fried carbs, real sugar—these are some of the nutritional components of a cheat meal.

Eat to Live

By committing to the Hot Mommy Next Door Eating Guidelines you will begin eating to live rather than living to eat. Your thoughts on food will transform as will your body. You will no longer think about what would be yummy right now. In stead you'll think about what your body requires to run efficiently and look good.

Timing

You should eat every three hours, so you'll need to be prepared. The timing of your first meal depends on a few factors such as when you plan to start and finish your workout and what else you need to accomplish that day (doctor's appointments, meetings, errands, work, and so on). You need to plan ahead to stay disciplined. Nobody gets into shape by accident. They work for it and at it.

If you are a stay-at-home mom who works out in the morning, your eating schedule may look as follows.

Sample Menu Items

Meal	Consumption Time	Dictated By
Breakfast	8:30 AM	9:30 AM SPIN® Class followed by weight training
Midmorning Snack	11:30 AM	Immediately following workout
Lunch	2:30 PM	Running errands after gym; before baby's afternoon nap
Midafternoon Snack	4:30 PM	In the middle of baby's play date or mom's social time
Dinner	7:30 PM	After baby is in bed but in time to watch your favorite TV show while folding laundry

If you are a mom who works outside the home, your eating schedule may look as follows.

Meal	Consumption Time	Dictated By
Breakfast	8:00 AM	Eating in the car while en route to drop off baby before heading to work for a 9:00 AM arrival time
Midmorning Snack	10:30 AM	During break time at work
Lunch	1:00 PM	Lunch meeting with colleagues
Midafternoon Snack	3:30 PM	Quickly at desk before 3:45 PM meeting
Dinner	6:00 PM	Allows for time to digest before heading to gym or in-home work-out at 7 PM

The Hot Mommy Next Door

In the beginning, keep your menus simple. Once you get used to this new way of eating, you will be able to get a little more creative.

Learn to Be Creative

Soon you will get a feel for the combinations of foods that work for your unique caloric and protein requirements. If you look at the breakfast and lunch recipes, you'll see similarities between them no matter what the food items are. So you can decide what you're in the mood for and then create a meal plan based on your personal nutritional needs.

This eating plan works because it is not technical, time consuming, or based on gimmicks. Instead it is based on basic nutritional principles. You can easily make smart choices based on the limited combinations of good, nutritious foods listed in this book.

And as you get familiar with the Smart Choices Eating Guidelines, feel free to creatively mix and match.

It was much harder for me to decide what I wanted to eat when I didn't eat as healthfully as I do now because I saw bad choices everywhere I looked. With my new "fit fast-food" eating style, I can easily make smart choices, prepare food quickly, and eat on the go. Most importantly, all the choices I make are healthy.

The next chapter will discuss real-world success strategies for your healthy new lifestyle.

Sample Menu Items

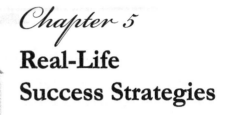

Chapter 5
Real-Life
Success Strategies

*T*o succeed on any weight loss and fitness program you must make a commitment to yourself. You can have all the knowledge in the world about nutrition and exercise, but unless you commit to becoming the best you that you can be, it won't happen. You must have the desire to change. Then you'll be able to follow a plan that gives you great results—a plan that prepares you to handle challenges.

Many moms come up to me and ask how I got back in shape so fast. But when I tell them the steps I took, some say, "Oh well, I like to eat yummy food too much to do that," or, "I couldn't find the time to make five meals like you do." This attitude sets them up for failure.

As I listen to them make excuses, I always think silently to myself that when they are ready to commit to themselves they'll have the body that they desire. Until then, it won't be possible. I cannot persuade them; their conviction must come from deep within.

You can't want something and not work for it. Those who tell you otherwise are blowing smoke up your skirt. But why wouldn't you want to work hard to be the best that you can be? Can you honestly say that you don't have time to feel good or take care of yourself? Try saying that out loud. It sounds pretty silly, doesn't it?

We wear many hats: wife, mother, chef, personal shopper, accountant, mechanic, cleaning service, sister, daughter, aunt, and lover just to name a few. How efficiently and happily can we function in all of those roles carrying extra baby weight? When we feel that we look good our confidence and self-esteem soar, which can affect many aspects of our lives. Being fit provides us with the energy to be active with our kids and accomplish all that we have on our plates every day as moms.

In this chapter, you'll learn simple strategies that will help you succeed using the Hot Mommy Next Door Program. These ten tips suit the real lifestyle of a woman taking care of small children.

Tip One: Make a Game Plan and Stick to It

In order to succeed in making smart choices, you must have a game plan. You need to know when, what, and where your next meal will come from. If you aren't prepared, you may fall off the wagon, because—believe me—once you start eating five small meals a day your body will anticipate its next meal, and you'll be cranky until you feed your belly. If you are prepared, you can avoid making bad food choices and stay disciplined.

Knowing what five clean meals you will be eating helps you to plan ahead if you have a doctor's appointment, play date, or business meeting.

Discipline, preparedness, and organization are crucial to your success. There are twenty-four hours in a day, and you only spend one or two of them at the gym. Adhering to the eating guidelines is the major predictor of your ability to succeed.

If you don't already use a day planner or calendar, get one and start writing down your activities and your children's. Make sure to review your planner or calendar nightly (after dinner or before bed) to remind you of any scheduled appointments or errands the next day. Make a game plan for success for the following day.

Tip Two: Stock Your Pantry

As moms, we are all a little short on time. If only the day was eight hours longer and there were two of us. Wishful thinking, I know! One way to make things simpler for ourselves is to schedule a weekly shopping excursion to stock up on exactly what we need to succeed on the program. I like to make my shopping list on Sundays after checking my handy dandy weekly planner and thinking about my gym schedule. Some of you have a work schedule to consider as well and will need to shop around your business hours.

Think about the week ahead and consider the following factors: Take stock of what you have food and beverage–wise and determine how long your current supplies will last you. Maybe a trip to the supermarket won't be absolutely necessary until Tuesday. Also, consider your schedule. Maybe it is easier for you to escape from the house solo on Sunday afternoon while your hubby tends to the kids, which will free up your Tuesday for another mom duty and allow you to shop whine free.

Another way to save time is to decide your weekly dinner menu in advance. Also, be sure to keep a shopping list at arm's reach in the kitchen. That way, when you run out of something or think of something you need or want, you can jot it down and you won't forget it. A magnetic pad that hangs on the

Real-Life Success Strategies

refrigerator door is a great device for this. When you're ready to go, you just rip the top sheet off the pad and you're on your way. Knowing exactly what you are shopping for will save you valuable time.

You could also use the shopping list at the back of the book (see page 131), and sign up for the downloadable version at www.thehmnd.com.

Tip Three: Stock a Go Bag

Now don't start moaning and groaning that you don't have time to eat or make five small meals a day because of course you do! As a mom of small kids—or big kids, for that matter—preparing meals might seem like all you do.

Let's take a look for a moment at how we feed our kids, our small kids that is. The day usually starts out with breakfast, followed by a midmorning snack and juice. Next comes lunch, followed up by a midafternoon snack and drink, and finally dinner for our little munchkins. Oh my, let's see … that's one, two, three, four, *five* meals, isn't it?

The key to staying on track is being prepared. As the mother of two small children, I never leave the house empty handed. I pack sippy cups, juice boxes, snack bags, snack cups, and so on to bring with me everywhere I go. You would never think of leaving the house empty handed and letting your little ones go snackless and thirsty, would you? The same goes for you!

Of course, as a mom of two small children, I understand how hectic things can get when you are trying to get out of the house and remember the arsenal of items required for your outing with kids in tow. Many times I leave the house with everything that my kids need and somehow manage to forget my snack, my workout towel, my head, and so forth on the counter where it will do me absolutely no good.

Throw into the mix the initial learning curve for the discipline and routine required of the Smart Choices Eating Guidelines, and it will more than likely take a little bit of time before you get into a groove.

This is where Plan B comes into play. What is Plan B you ask? Plan B consists of knowing exactly where you can purchase, for example, your protein bar of choice (since yours is in the pantry where you left it, and you have a play date to go to after the gym). Whether that location is the drug store, nutrition store, or grocery store, you need to know where you can get an allowable snack to hold you over until you get home for lunch.

Also, it might be a good idea to keep a stash of almonds preportioned into individual servings in your glove compartment to carry you through such an emergency. That way you can avoid the danger that you'll make a poor choice if you have a sudden craving and no supplies on hand. Organizational skills are key factors to success; you will master them with practice.

If you will be on the go for part of the day, pack your snacks and meals and bring them with you. You need to consume calories on a regular timetable to have the energy to take care of your little ones properly. We all know that being a good mom means taking care of your own needs first: physically, mentally, emotionally, spiritually, and nutritionally.

Tip Four: Keep "Tricks of the Trade" in Your Car

Success is all about being prepared ladies, so let's talk more about on-the-go preparedness. As moms we spend a lot of time in the car taking the little ones here and there. Therefore, in addition to your go bag, you must stock your car appropriately with drinks and snacks. I like to think of these items, which may or may not also be found in your go bag, as my "tricks of the trade," my favorite supplies that aren't always readily available.

I always have a water bottle or two on hand and an assortment of individual sugar-free drink packets. If I want flavor in my water, I can empty a sugar-free drink packet into a twenty-four-ounce sports bottle and shake it up for a delicious treat of my choice. This comes in handy when I am eating my lunch on the go, which is more often than not. Whether picking up my favorite wrap or eating one of my own concoctions, I always have a drink available.

Real-Life Success Strategies

It's also a good idea to carry sugarless gum in the automobile. In my car there's always a pack or two sitting on my dashboard for when I need to divert my attention from a craving. Whenever I feel the need to chomp on something or I'm thinking about chocolate way too much, I just pop a piece of gum in my mouth. I view it as a dessert of sorts.

Finally, when I am in the mood for a little treat and hit the drive-thru for a cup of decaf coffee or tea, I have handy my own nondairy creamer and individual Splenda flavor blend sticks. I confess, my glove compartment looks like a mini-mart.

Tip Five: Measure Up

After a while, you'll become a pro at determining what four ounces of sliced turkey looks and feels like, but in the beginning a scale can help you measure portion sizes. They are inexpensive, readily available (lots of times you can even find them in your local grocery store), and very practical for your purposes.

Scales can be a real time saver. For instance, you can figure out how many spirals of fusilli or sticks of spaghetti add up to a two-ounce serving. Then divide the contents of the box into individual servings and bag them up for later use. If you take time in the beginning to measure portions, you will save time later!

Another easy way to determine portion size is to learn to eyeball them based on everyday equivalents. For your convenience, I have listed equivalents for common portion sizes on next page.

The Hot Mommy Next Door

General Equivalents

1 Cup	A baseball or small fist
1/2 Cup	Half a baseball
2/3 Cup	A tennis ball
1 Teaspoon	A thumb tip (Tip of thumb to first joint)
1 Tablespoon	3 thumb tips or one thumb
1 Medium fruit	A baseball
1 Medium potato	A tennis ball
3 ounces of meat, fish, or poultry	A deck of cards, palm of your hand, or computer mouse
1 ounce of nuts	A ping-pong ball
1/2 Cup berries/fruit	A cupped handful

Tip Six: Overcoming Carb Cravings

You may not consider dinner complete without a side dish of carbs. Whether it is macaroni and cheese, french fries, or rice, dinner is not dinner without them. While carbs may hit the spot after a tough day, they may well stick to that spot—and then you'll be in trouble.

Cutting carbs from the dinner menu takes some adjusting, especially with your increased workouts and the energy you spend chasing around a little one (or two, or three). Carbs are a great source of quick energy. Although the Smart Choices Eating Guidelines allow and even require appropriate carbohydrate consumption early in the day, you may still long for extra carbs. By the time you arrive at your fifth and last meal of the day you might be tempted to resort back to your old eating habits.

Luckily, soon your body, mind, and stomach will adjust to tapering off carbs in the afternoon. But pesky cravings will creep out of the woodwork from time to time, and you need a plan for handling them.

Real-Life Success Strategies

In order to satiate my occasional nighttime carb craving, I turn to one of the following: a low-carb wheat wrap (3 grams net carbs and 50 calories), a small handful of brown rice (less than half of a serving, more like a quarter serving; this is a purely mental solution), or a small handful of low-carb cereal (same deal as the rice).

If I believe a wrap will do the trick that evening, I'll fill one up with my veggies of the night and chow down. Maybe I'll even add a sprinkle of fat-free cheese.

If a wrap just won't cut it, I will eat a small portion of brown rice. I resort to this tactic when I am desperate due to the fact that "Aunt Flo" has come to town or I had an unusually active day. Sometimes I eat my new favorite low-carb pasta instead of the rice. Yes, it exists and you can find it in my list of Favorites By Brand (see page 135).

My husband is not always on the same page as I am when it comes to tapering carbs at dinner time. Unfortunately for him, he has no choice but to eat a healthy, low-carb dinner because I refuse to be a cafeteria. We all eat the same food items. However, he does occasionally request a carb-infused meal, and I sometimes accede to his request. Let's say grilled chicken and stir-fry vegetables are on the menu for the evening, but your other half wants some pasta. In this case, just prepare the regularly scheduled meal right along with low-carb pasta. Your husband gets his spaghetti and you allow yourself a controlled, measured portion of low-carb pasta (remember to use your scale to measure dry pasta) to satiate your craving. Remember low-carb pasta still has calories so you don't want to overeat.

When I do this, I place a little pasta in a bowl and then throw my veggies and chicken on top, or just eat the pasta as a side dish with a spray or two of imitation butter and a sprinkle of parmesan cheese.

You may also opt to make turkey meatballs (see recipe on page 76). Then add the vegetable of your choice to the pasta and pretend you are going out on the town. If you use sauce, make sure it has low-sugar and low-sodium content. Otherwise, skip the sauce and resort to the imitation butter spray and a sprinkle of parmesan cheese.

I have also learned frequently a handful of low-carb cereal while I'm cooking will kill my carb craving before it gets the best of me. The cereal trick also works during the day if you acquire a case of the munchies between meals.

Tip Seven: Sweet Tooth Survival

Now, let me remind all you sweetaholic and chocoholic ladies of my dessert advice from Chapter Three: Jell-O Sugar Free Low Calorie Gelatin Snacks containing 0 sugars and 10 calories should be your new best friend.

However, desperate times may call for desperate measures, and when chocolate cravings present themselves, I have been known to resort to other measures. A quarter of a chocolate-flavored protein bar, for example, is a better alternative than the real thing.

Or you can follow this recipe for Fake Brownies:

Real-Life Success Strategies

Fake Brownies

Ingredients

1 chocolate flavored high-protein, low-carb meal-replacement shake

1 packet of plain instant oatmeal

1/2 cup egg whites

Nonstick cooking spray

Instructions

Mix the meal-replacement shake with the oatmeal and egg whites. Spray an 8" x 8" inch pan with a nonstick cooking spray. Pour the batter into pan and bake at 350 degrees for 15–20 minutes.

Be careful about the time of day you eat this treat. The oatmeal packet and the shake both contain carbs and calories, which you need to count in addition to your regular meals. You don't want to overeat.

In other words, monitor your portions and beware of when you consume them.

It is important to mention that these "fake" brownies have a short shelf life, so you may want to consider sharing them with a friend or cutting the recipe in half!

My last craving trick is a sugar-free Fudgsicle sweetened with Splenda, which contains 35 calories and 3.5 carbs per bar. I recommend saving this option for emergencies because it may open Pandora's box.

Sweetaholics are in luck. Even if you have one Jell-O Sugar Free Low Calorie Gelatin Snack Cup after lunch and another after dinner that only equal twenty calories. You may also opt to buy sugar free Popsicles (10 calories and 1 net carb), Creamsicles (20 calories and 2 net carbs), or a variety pack containing both plus the Fudgsicles mentioned above.

Some product labels list total carbohydrates as the amount of carbs per bar, but the carb counts I have listed here are the total carbohydrates minus the dietary fiber and sugar alcohols.

There are also numerous brands of sugar-free lollipops on the market that contain zero carbs and minimal calories. Try those to curb your cravings.

If you do your homework, you'll find acceptable replacements that satisfy your sweet tooth.

Keep in mind that you should not use these tricks daily because you don't want to become dependent on them. These are in case of emergencies. You should only resort to these tricks as a safety net to avoid pure disaster.

Real-Life Success Strategies

Tip Eight: Analyze Your Slips

Another key to stay on track is to recognize when you tend to eat the wrong things and why. With awareness, you might be able to prevent an episode of binge eating. For example, I am an emotional eater. When I am feeling down and I've had one of those days, a Big Mac and McFlurry sound pretty appealing to me.

The old me would have succumbed to temptation and partaken in the instant gratification of the greasy, fatty yumminess of the "golden arches." The new me, however, can take a step back and recognize that a moment of weakness is about to occur, and she understands why.

It's an opportunity.

With awareness, I can remind myself that if I indulge I will only feel better for an instant. Also, that I might feel guilty and spiral into a deeper depression if I give in to my temporary insanity. In addition, I remind myself of the cheat meal and dessert that I allow myself once a week. Taking a minute to daydream about the succulent treat my tongue plans to enjoy enables me to stay on track.

Tip Nine: Praise Yourself

It takes a lot of discipline and commitment to stay on track with an eating and fitness plan and to make the right choices. In today's world, industry-generated conveniences make it easier and more convenient to travel down a less healthy path. You should be proud when you resist.

Think of the energy, time, and planning it takes you to make exercise a part of your day. Make sure to pat yourself on the back for a job well done. You deserve high praise and kudos for taking charge of your health and wellness.

Tip Ten: Take a Moment for Yourself

Although this may sound like an oxymoron when you have small children, it's good advice. You have to reserve time for yourself. Seize a moment whenever the opportunity presents itself. Steal a moment even if it doesn't! Yes, this may be easier said then done once a newborn enters your home, but after you figure out your routine—and you will—you need to build some "me" time into it.

We all need time to regroup and relax, even if only for a moment, to get our heads together so we don't entirely lose ourselves in motherhood. Don't forget, you are still an individual with needs and, let's face it … we each have to look out for our own well-being.

I think of the gym as my shining opportunity to take care of myself mentally and physically. But I've also added a spiritual component to my morning: before starting my gym routine, I tune out the world and tune into myself by listening to a song of my choice on my iPod. This allows me to check in with myself after the bustle of the morning and to ground myself for the rest of the day ahead.

Nothing relaxes me and allows me to continue my routine like taking a few deep, focused breaths.

In the next chapter, we'll talk about exercise. Working out on a near-daily basis is a key component of the Hot Mommy Next Door Program. It's also a lot of fun and a great way to show yourself love and attention. Fit moms make better mothers because they are strong, happy, and energetic. So, ladies, turn the page and get ready to have some fun.

Chapter 6

Make Your Workout Count

I've said it before and I'll say it again: anything worth having is worth working for ("work" being the operative word), which brings me to the exercise portion of the Hot Mommy Next Door guidelines. Let's talk about good, old-fashioned exercise. This aspect of the program will accelerate your weight loss more than cutting calories alone.

I would love to say that you can look fit and fabulous without lifting a finger or breaking a sweat. Maybe you could lose weight by ingesting a magic pill or by using a space-aged, Jetson-like machine (George Jetson, that is) that leaves you looking flawless. Sorry to disappoint. It isn't called a workout for the heck of it. Exercise actually requires discipline and determination. But the good news is that you're probably going to like it once you get used to it. You might even get addicted like I did.

Please don't let a fear of exercise deter you. Your workout will help you become the best you possible. Imagine if you had passed up the opportunity to have a baby because of the physical effort and sacrifices it requires: Forty weeks where your body doesn't belong to you and then the actual labor and birthing process. *Ouch!* And let's not forget the lifetime commitment and worry that accompany motherhood. If you had let fear hold you back, you would be missing out on the most miraculous journey of your life.

Since you are already doing the hardest—and most rewarding—job in the world, why not also look and feel your best doing it? When you work out on a regular basis, your energy level skyrockets, your body tones and tightens, and your clothes fit better, all of which naturally boost your confidence and self-esteem. That makes you a more available mother, one who can enjoy her family. An added bonus: it will improve your sex life!

If you're already familiar with exercise and love to work out, you are one step ahead of the game. I would bet that you're itching to get back into your routine so you can regain the svelte body you once knew. I want to assure you that your body will go back to feeling normal again in time. It only takes a few workouts to break the ice and reintroduce your body to an exercise routine. Then you're on your way. Soon you'll have built up your fitness base, and you'll feel like your old self once more. Muscles have memory, so your body will literally welcome the workout regimen like a long lost friend. If you happen to be a novice to exercise, don't worry. Read on to learn how to get started.

In this chapter I'm going to introduce you to your two new best buddies: cardiovascular exercise and weight training. The key to a successful exercise regimen is the combination of these two activities. While eating right is a major factor in dropping unwanted baby weight, cardiovascular exercise is crucial to reaching your higher-level fitness goals. Add weight training to the mix, and you will transform and sculpt your body by replacing fat with muscle. More importantly, you'll take pleasure in the aesthetic effects you achieve, and you'll be healthier.

As always, consult a doctor before heading to the gym to work out after recently having a baby.

Cardiovascular Program

Let's address the cardiovascular portion of the Hot Mommy workout first. Cardiovascular exercise is a great way to burn calories, increase blood and oxygen circulation, build your endurance, and improve the health of your heart. To make the most of your cardiovascular workout, take four factors into consideration: frequency, duration, variation, and intensity.

Frequency: As you strive to reach your prepregnancy weight, I would recommend at least five if not six cardio workouts per week. The idea is to "shock" your body until you reach one or two of your goals. You most likely did little exercise between the final month of your pregnancy (or longer if exercise was not on your pregnancy agenda) and at least six weeks postpartum. Now the idea is to get your body moving and often.

Duration: Make sure your cardiovascular activities range from thirty to forty-five minutes. Pick a pace that is challenging but sustainable for the minimum thirty-minute requirement. In order to see results from cardiovascular exercise, you need to keep your heart rate up long enough to tap into your fat stores.

When you work out, your body first burns stored carbohydrates. While you benefit from the calories you burn while working through your stored carbohydrates, you want to get to the point where you're burning as much fat as possible. If you do your weight training first, you will boost your heart rate. By increasing your heart rate, you start your cardio routine one step closer to fighting the fat.

Remember always to factor warm-up and cool-down routines into your workouts for safety.

Real-Life Success Strategies

Variation: I suggest alternating between three different types of cardio activities every week. It is important to change things up so that your body doesn't adapt to a particular workout thus causing your weight loss progress to level off because your body no longer responds to the same old routine. Varying your routine will ensure results and keep you from getting bored.

When I first returned to the gym after my second child was born, I did whatever it took. I was on a mission. One day I would get on the treadmill and run for thirty minutes, the next day I would take a SPIN® class that lasted from forty-five minutes to an hour, and the day after that I would get on the Stairmaster for at least thirty minutes. I became such a fanatic of the SPIN® program that I got certified as an instructor and now teach classes myself.

Cardio Options

Walking (briskly)	Dancing	Bicycling
Jogging	Aerobics	Tennis
Stair Climbing	Stepping	Racquetball
Revolving Stair Climbing	Skiing	Swimming
Elliptical Training	Ice Skating	Canoeing
SPINNING®	Rollerblading	Rowing
Kickboxing	Roller Skating	Jumping rope

Levels of Intensity: In order to benefit from your cardiovascular workouts, you need to work out at the right level of intensity. A good rule of thumb is to exercise at a level where it is difficult to carry on a conversation. Short sentences are okay, such as, "The baby cried all night," "Very tired," "He's a jerk" (he being your husband), or "Can't talk right now," but no more. We aren't chilling out, ladies. We are working out!

You could also use a heart rate monitor to gage the level of intensity of your workout. Go online, to the library, or to a well-staffed sporting goods store to find out more about them. These monitors are great tools because they provide you with continuous and accurate heart rate measurements throughout the duration of your workout. This allows you to pace yourself and to work in the ideal zone of intensity for weight loss, which is different for every person. This is known as your target heart rate. You can determine your target heart rate via the Internet. I recommend you type in the key words "target heart rate calculator" to be directed to numerous sites that offer this free service. Or you could just use the aforementioned speaking guideline. Whatever your heart desires!

Remember, you can control the intensity of the machines you work out on. Even if you think a certain machine such as the Stairmaster is the devil in disguise, try it out. Pick a level that is challenging but doable. This will help you build up your strength and endurance. Then you can take it up a notch.

If you choose to take a group fitness class, the same holds true: you are in control of the level of intensity at which you execute the class. In the beginning your level of exertion will most likely differ from the veterans in the class, but that doesn't mean that you won't get a great workout. In time, as you build up your strength and endurance, you will be able to take it to the next level. The idea is to challenge yourself and get results.

If you opt to take a group fitness class to fulfill your cardio requirements, make sure that you choose the class wisely. Yoga, while enjoyable and beneficial, does not consistently elevate your heart rate in the way an interval step class would. Your goal is to challenge your heart.

Once you achieve one or two of your fitness goals, you can experiment with different classes. For now, keep your eye on the prize—your hot body!

Final Thoughts on Cardio

You're not always going to like your cardio regimen, but music does wonders to boost a cardio workout. You will quickly discover which methods of cardio you prefer and which you dread, but you must persevere through them all to

Real-Life Success Strategies

reach your goals.

Running is my least favorite cardio activity, although I know many people who love to run. Nonetheless, I did it every week when I was dropping my baby weight in order to reach my initial goals. SPINNING® is my favorite cardio activity, and it is hard for me not to do at least four classes in a week. Keep working out, and you will find your groove.

Many of you may be new to the world of working out, and even if you are not, you will most likely have to slowly build up your strength and endurance when returning to the gym after giving birth to a human being. You can expect to feel a little bit sore a day or two after an intense workout. Muscles "burn" when they are fatigued, and they are sore during recovery. Always be sure to rest one day a week to give your body a chance to restore itself.

It is essential to listen to your body and pay attention to your level of exertion. You need to challenge yourself, but don't go overboard. Your body will tell you when you are able to take it up a notch and move on to the next level.

Weight Training Program

The second key element in our weight loss and optimal fitness program is weight training. The great thing about weight training is that it raises your body's metabolic rate, so you continue to burn calories after you stop working out, even while at rest. Pretty cool, huh? This differs from the cardiovascular workout because cardio burns calories only for the duration of the workout.

Weight training is the key to transforming the shape of your body. Through lifting weights your body replaces fat with muscle, giving you muscle tone and definition as well as a lean appearance. This is why the combination of both weight training and cardiovascular training is essential to a successful exercise program.

Many of you may have steered clear of weight training in the past out of a fear of becoming big and bulky. I would like to put that fear to rest right now. Because of our low testosterone levels, women cannot produce large, bulky muscles like men do. Nonetheless, weight training will improve your muscle tone and strength while it does away with fatty tissue.

Before you start your weight training, it's a good idea to warm up with five minutes of easy cardio (perhaps a brisk walk on the treadmill), and to do some simple stretching of the hamstrings, the quadriceps, the biceps, the triceps—in fact, you should stretch the whole kit and caboodle. Hold each stretch for twenty to thirty seconds without bouncing. You want to get the blood circulating in your muscles so the fibers are more flexible. This helps avoid injury and prevents soreness. You may choose to stretch between sets as well.

Choose a weight to lift that's heavy enough to challenge you, yet one that you can manage to lift for fifteen to twenty repetitions. Doing this high a number of repetitions of each movement will help you achieve the look you desire.

I am fortunate to be able to work out first thing in the morning. Did I say first thing? Well, first thing *after* I feed the kids, get them dressed, brush their teeth, pack their snacks and lunches, change a diaper or two, facilitate a trip to the potty, grab toys for the car, referee fights, and drop my kids off at school.

Working out in the morning energizes me for the rest of the day. It definitely is a form of therapy for me. And any time I have to skip a day, I really feel the difference in my mood and my energy level.

My personal weight regimen involves five weight-training sessions over the course of the workweek (Monday through Friday) divided as follows:

- Monday: shoulders.
- Tuesday: legs (quadriceps, hamstrings, and calves).
- Wednesday: back (upper and lower).

123

- Thursday: chest and triceps.
- Friday: biceps.
- Weekend: rest.

I also target my abdominal muscles: upper, middle, lower, and side. Incorporate abs into your workout routine either by doing a series of crunches to target each section or by taking an abdominals class three to four times a week (every other day).

I do this weight training in addition to my six cardiovascular training sessions per week. But if you feel "crunched" for time, you might choose a different combination of activities for your regimen, perhaps targeting your muscle groups three days a week rather than five. Whatever your schedule or time constraints may be, you can tailor a program that fits into your life.

Ten Major Muscle Groups

Upper Body	Lower Body	Arms	Waist
Deltoids (Shoulders)	Quadriceps (Front of Legs)	Biceps (Front of Arms)	Abdominals
Pectorals (Chest)	Hamstrings (Back of Legs)	Triceps (Back of Arms)	Lower Back
Laterals (Upper Back)	Calves		

The key to efficient weight training is knowledge. Those of you who choose to hire a trainer as I did will have an advantage over those of you who don't. A trainer will complete your body composition analysis (see instructions on page 11), evaluate your body mass (see page 13), devise a workout routine for you based on your goals, and walk you through it until you are familiar with the exercises. The rest is up to you.

If continuous training sessions don't fit into your budget, perhaps you can splurge on one to three sessions to complete the BCA, learn about the different muscle groups, and learn to work targeted muscles properly.

Those of you who belong to a gym—or intend to join one—but opt not to hire a trainer may benefit from taking a gym orientation session. A gym orientation normally consists of a guided tour of the gym by a fitness trainer. Your escort will introduce you to the various machines, explain what muscle group each machine targets, and teach you how to adjust and operate it.

Those of you who intend to workout at home need to find another way to learn to work your target muscle groups. You'll need free weights and a book or fitness magazine with good illustrations, or a video program to get you started.

It's easiest to learn if someone teaches you because you can ask questions. But while trainers are convenient, you don't need a trainer to be successful. We live in an age of abundant instructional resources including the Internet, fitness magazines, books, videos, and cable television shows, so you can definitely construct a program on your own by doing a little bit of research.

Going Solo or Going with a Friend?

It is great if you have a workout partner to motivate you, chit chat with you, and hopefully challenge you. However, I believe the biggest mistake some women make is to rely too heavily on their friends and let their presence or absence dictate whether or not they workout.

What happens when your friend calls you at 7:00 A.M. (because she knows you're a mom and it's not too early to be calling as you've probably been up for at least half an hour already) to tell you that she's not feeling well or her little one has a runny nose so she won't be able to join you for the workout today?

Real-Life Success Strategies

If you have accustomed yourself to depending on a friend's presence to motivate you to workout, your answer might be that you don't work out that day. *Bzzzz!* I am here to tell you that this is the wrong answer!

I cannot stress this enough: the only way you will ever achieve your goals and the body that you desire is to depend on yourself and yourself alone. This is your journey, your body, and your life. You are in the driver's seat. So, while it is okay to have a workout partner, don't let her absence get in the way of achieving your hot "mamalicious" body.

Making It Count

You must be committed to yourself and the process in order to see the results you've always wanted but perhaps haven't been able to attain. You need to see past your limitations. Trust that the body you desire can be yours. You can look that good. But only you can make it happen.

The key to success is to push yourself. You need to ask, "Am I doing my personal best or could I up the ante a little more?" If you can carry on a conversation while doing your cardio, I have news for you: you are not working hard enough. If you're not panting and perspiring, it's the same deal. You need to work as hard as you can for half an hour of cardio or a sufficient number of reps of weights. Always be honest with yourself. After all, you will be the one to benefit.

My workout motto is "Make it count." Why go to the gym if you are not going to work hard enough? Walking through the gym doors does not constitute a workout. You have to go and take what is yours.

Remember, ladies, if you ever see a woman with a body you admire at the gym or anywhere else for that matter, it is probably not due to her genetic heritage (although we would love to believe that). It is because she works hard for her fitness and makes smart choices.

Knowledge is power. And now that you have the tools to design a highly effective workout regimen, you can become the best you that you can be. We all have personal limitations, genetic predispositions, and different body types, but we can will ourselves to have the best bodies we can.

The Hot Mommy Next Door Program is not a fad, a diet, or something we do only until we lose our baby weight. It is a terrific lifestyle that boosts energy, keeps us fit and healthy, and increases our confidence in every way. It is a way of living based on making good, smart choices.

Remember to make it count!

Real-Life Success Strategies

Afterword
The Big Picture

Being a Hot Mommy Next Door isn't all about appearances, ladies. (Shhh, don't tell anyone I said that.) There is a bigger picture to address. This lifestyle is about developing healthy habits: setting a good example regarding food consumption and physical activity for our children as well as maintaining good health so we can be around a long time for our families.

We live in a culture of excess and immediate gratification, and it is very easy to fall prey to these factors, which can lead to ill health. A healthy lifestyle is all about discipline and routines, which are great foundations that can carry over into other areas of our lives as well as the lives of our children.

Aside from the obvious benefits of working out and eating well such as reduced body weight, reduced body fat, and improved physical appearance, there are other less obvious benefits, including a reduced risk of disease, reduced instances of depression, reduced stress, better sleep, increased energy, improved self-esteem, and decreased blood pressure and cholesterol, just to name a few.

If you're not happy, you can't make the people who matter most to you happy. By making my health and fitness a priority over the last few years, I became a better mom, wife, daughter, sister, and friend. More important, my journey inspired me to write this book to help other moms like you be the best they can be and feel good about their bodies and minds.

So here you are, at this moment in your life, with this book in your hands, contemplating changing your lifestyle with The Hot Mommy Next Door Program. I hope you're feeling great about your decision to take control of your body, mind, and spirit. I am proud of you for taking the first steps, and I hope you are proud too. Those first steps may seem like the hardest but the rewards are immense.

I'm here to support you the rest of the way and I'd love to hear about your progress and success. Please keep in touch at feedback@thehmnd.com.

Alison's Shopping List

*O*kay, ladies. For your convenience, I've constructed a master shopping list to facilitate your weekly shopping trips. Simply check off the items you will need for the week ahead. You'll have to determine the quantity you need of each item depending on how many people you'll be cooking for. Perhaps, unbeknownst to him, your husband's eating lifestyle can change along with yours. Be sure to visit www.thehmnd.com and sign up to receive a free downloadable and reusable Hot Mommy Next Door shopping list.

Don't forget, just because an item is on the master list doesn't mean you need to purchase it every time you shop. One week you'll opt for whole-wheat English muffins, the next week whole-wheat mini bagels. Use the guidelines from the book to make wholesome, healthy choices.

Do you remember when I said that almost everything you need for your new eating lifestyle can be found on the outskirts of the grocery store? As you begin your next shopping excursion, pay attention to where your list takes you. If you find yourself in an aisle, note what you are selecting and then look around the rest of the aisle at what you are not selecting. It should be pretty clear why the aisles are bad news for the most part.

You could also compare a few nutritional labels. Look at the nutritional facts on the products you are selecting based on the smart choices eating guidelines and compare them to the labels of similar products (for example, your plain oatmeal versus a banana nut-flavored oatmeal). Note the differences and similarities between the products. This knowledge will empower you to continue making smart choices later on.

You can find most (probably all) of the products on this list at your local grocery stores, nutrition markets, and big box retailers. If you are unable to find a product or if the price tag is too high at your local stores, I recommend searching on the Internet for the product at a lower price. This is especially helpful for meal-replacement shakes. A little bit of research can go a long way in saving you money.

Now, go have fun and do what you do best: shopping!

SHOPPING LIST

WHOLE GRAINS
BREADS:
__ 100% Whole Wheat Bread
__ 100% Whole Wheat Bagels or Mini Bagels
__ 100% Whole Wheat English Muffins
__ 100% Whole Wheat Pita Bread
__ 100% Whole Wheat Tortillas/Wraps
__ 100% Whole Wheat Low-Carb and Low-Fat
Tortillas
__ Sprouted 100% Whole-Grain Bread
__ 100% Whole Wheat Crackers

PASTA:
__ 100% Whole Wheat Pasta
__ Low-Carb Pasta

RICE:
__ Minute Instant Brown Rice
__ Brown Rice Cakes, Lightly Salted
__ Wild Rice

CEREAL:
__ 100% Whole Grain Cereal
__ Instant Oatmeal Packets, Plain

VEGETABLES
FRESH:
__ Asparagus
__ Bell Pepper (Red/Green)
__ Broccoli
__ Brussels Sprouts
__ Carrots
__ Corn
__ Green Beans
__ Mushrooms
__ Onions (Red/White/Yellow)
__ Romaine Lettuce
__ Spinach
__ Squash
__ Sweet Potatoes
__ Zucchini

FROZEN:
__ Vegetable Medley
__ Stir Fry Vegetables

CANNED:
__ Corn (low sugar/low sodium)
__ Light Red Kidney Beans

FRUITS
FRESH:
__ Apples (Green/Red)
__ Avocadoes
__ Blueberries
__ Grapefruit
__ Grape Tomatoes
__ Pears
__ Peaches
__ Pineapple
__ Raspberries
__ Strawberries

FROZEN:
__ Blueberries (Unsweetened)
__ Pineapple (Unsweetened)
__ Raspberries (Unsweetened)
__ Strawberries (Unsweetened)

CANNED:
__ Diced Tomatoes (no salt added)

LEAN CUTS OF MEAT
CHICKEN:
__ Boneless Skinless Chicken Breast
__ Boneless Skinless Chicken Tenderloins
__ Boneless Skinless Chicken Cutlets
__ Rotisserie Chicken
__ Roasted Chicken Breast Slices from Deli, Low
Sodium
__ Canned Chicken, All White in Water

TURKEY:
__ Lean Ground Turkey, (no more than 7% fat)
__ Lean Turkey Burgers, Frozen
__ Roasted Turkey Breast Slices from Deli, Low
Sodium

PORK:
__ Lean Pork Chops
__ Pork Tenderloin

RED MEAT:
___ Lean Ground Beef (4% fat)
___ Filet Mignon

FISH:
___ Tilapia
___ Salmon
___ Mahi Mahi
___ Canned Tuna, Solid White Albacore in Water

MEAL REPLACEMENTS AND SUPPLEMENTS

MEAL REPLACEMENTS:
___ High Protein Meal Replacement Shake Packets
___ Ready-to-Drink Meal Replacement Shakes
___ Protein Bars

SUPPLEMENTS:
___ 100% Whey Protein Powder
___ Ready-to-Drink Protein Shakes

MISCELLANEOUS

REFRIGERATED/DAIRY:
___ Cottage Cheese (2% Milk fat)
___ Yogurt Cups
___ Yogurt Smoothies
___ Soymilk, Light/Plain
___ Egg Whites
___ Egg Substitute
___ Fat Free Cheese Singles (Slices)
___ Fat Free Shredded Cheese

FROZEN:
___ Veggie Burgers

PRODUCE:
___ Raw Almonds

BEVERAGES

WATER:
___ Twenty-four-ounce Sports Water Bottles
___ One-Gallon Jugs

SUGAR-FREE DRINK MIXES:
___ Two-quart mixers
___ Multi-Serve Bottles (Ready-To-Drink)
___ Single Serve Bottles (Ready-To-Drink)
___ Travel Packets (Single Servings)

CARBONATED:
___ Sparkling Natural Mineral Water
      (plain or flavored)
___ Diet Soft Drink (Clear), Caffeine, Sugar, and
      Carb Free

COFFEE/TEA:
___ Decaffeinated Coffee (Your Favorite)
___ Decaffeinated Tea (Your Favorite)

CONDIMENTS/SEASONINGS/SPICES
___ Mustard (plain)
___ Ketchup (Low Carb/Low Sugar)
___ Parmesan Cheese (Regular or Fat Free)
___ Mayonnaise (Light/Reduced Fat/Fat Free)
___ Tomato Sauce
      (No Added Sugar/Low Sugar and Low Carb)
___ Imitation Butter Spray
___ Non-Dairy Creamer
___ Balsamic Vinegar
___ Salad Dressing
___ Lemon Juice
___ Worcestershire Sauce
___ Peanut Butter (Reduced Sugar, Low Sodium)
___ No Calorie Sweetener, Individual Packets
___ Sugar-Free Flavor Blends for Coffee,
      Individual Sticks
___ Sugar-Free Jelly/Preserves
___ Sugar-Free Syrup
___ Almond Slices
___ Fresh Garlic
___ Fresh Salsa
___ Fresh Hummus
___ Chili Seasoning (Low Sodium)
___ Salt-Free Seasoning Blends
___ Any Salt-Free Season
      (Ex. Garlic Powder/Pepper/Oregano)
___ Any Salt-Free Spice (Ex. Cinnamon or Nutmeg)

OILS/COOKING SPRAYS
___ Extra Virgin Olive Oil
___ Canola Oil
___ Non-Stick Cooking Spray

DESSERTS
___ Sugar-Free Gelatin
___ Fat Free Dairy Whipped Topping
___ Sugar-Free Popsicles, Creamsicles, Fudgsicles
___ Sugar-Free Gum

Alison's Favorite Brands

*F*or your benefit, I have detailed a list of my favorite products, which have contributed enormously to the success of my healthy lifestyle. Having these or similar products on hand is crucial to eating well and reaching your fitness goals. They will equip you to make smart eating choices when you feel hungry and it's time for a meal.

FAVORITES BY BRAND

WHOLE GRAINS

BREAD:

- ☐ Nature's Own 100% Whole-wheat Bread
- ☐ Lender's 100% Whole-wheat Bagels
- ☐ Pepperidge Farm 100% Whole-wheat Mini Bagels
- ☐ Tam-X-icos White Corn Tortillas
- ☐ La Tortilla Factory Whole-wheat Low-carb/ Low-fat Tortillas, Original
- ☐ La Banderita Low Carb Low Fat Soft Taco
- ☐ Ezekiel 4:9 Organic Sprouted 100% Whole-grain Flourless Bread
- ☐ Ok-mok 100% Whole of the Wheat Stone Ground Sesame Crackers

PASTA:

- ☐ Gia Russa Whole-wheat pastas
- ☐ Dreamfields Healthy Carb Living Pasta

RICE:

- ☐ Kraft Minute Instant Whole-grain Brown Rice
- ☐ Birds Eye Steamfresh Whole Grain Brown Rice
- ☐ Quaker Rice Cakes, Lightly Salted

CEREAL:

- ☐ Kashi 7 Whole-grain Puffs
- ☐ Nutritious Living Hi-Lo Cereal

VEGETABLES

FRESH:

- ☐ Dole, Fresh Express, or generic store brand Hearts of Romaine Lettuce (Ready-to-Eat)
- ☐ GreenLine Fresh Trimmed Green Beans, Microwavable in Bag
- ☐ Eat Smart Bagged Vegetable Mixes (Stir-Fry, Broccoli, Carrots and Cauliflower)

FROZEN:

- ☐ Birds Eye Steamfresh (Selects, Mixtures, and Singles)

CANNED:

- ☐ Green Giant Super Sweet Yellow and White Corn
- ☐ Bush's Best Light Red Kidney Beans

FRUITS

FROZEN:

- ☐ Dole Pineapple Chunks
- ☐ Dole Wild Blueberries
- ☐ Dole Whole Strawberries

LEAN CUTS OF MEAT

POULTRY:

FRESH

- ☐ Jennie-O Lean Ground Turkey Meat
- ☐ Jennie-O Extra Lean Ground Turkey Meat

FROZEN

- ☐ Jennie-O Turkey Burgers, Savory Seasoned or Plain (70% Less Fat)

DELI

- ☐ Boar's Head Golden Classic Oven Roasted Chicken Breast
- ☐ Boar's Head Ovengold Roast Breast of Turkey, Skinless or Lower Sodium Premium Turkey, Skinless

CANNED

- ☐ Valley Fresh, 98% Fat-Free, Premium Chunk White Chicken in Water

PORK:

FRESH

- ☐ Maverick Ranch Natural Pork, Lean Pork Chops

RED MEAT:

FRESH

- ☐ Maverick Ranch Naturalite Ground Beef (4%)
- ☐ Laura's Lean Ground Beef (4%)

FISH:

CANNED

- ☐ Starkist Solid White Albacore Tuna in Water

MEAL REPLACEMENTS AND SUPPLEMENTS

HIGH-PROTEIN LOW-CARB MEAL REPLACEMENT SHAKES

- ☐ Labrada, Lean Body for Her
- ☐ Labrada, Lean Body, Carbwatchers

READY-TO-DRINK MEAL REPLACEMENT SHAKES

- ☐ EAS Myoplex Lite

PROTEIN BARS

- ☐ Pure Protein

100% WHEY PROTEIN POWDER

- ☐ Optimum Nutrition (ON) 100% Whey
- ☐ Energy Athletics Strengths (EAS) 100% Whey Powder

READY-TO-DRINK PROTEIN SHAKES

- ☐ EAS Advantdge Carb Control RTD
- ☐ Pure Protein

FAVORITES BY BRAND

MISCELLANEOUS
REFRIGERATED/DAIRY:
- Breakstone's Live Active Cottage Cheese (plain, 2% milk fat)
- Dannon Light & Fit Carb & Sugar Control Yogurt Cups
- Dannon Light & Fit Carb & Sugar Control Smoothie
- 8th Continent Light Soymilk Original
- All Whites 100% Liquid Egg Whites
- Egg Beaters 99% Real Eggs
- Kraft Fat Free Singles (American)
- Kraft Free Shredded Cheddar or Mozzarella Cheese

FROZEN:
- Boca Meatless Burgers, All American Flame Grilled or Original (Vegan)
- Morning Star Farms (Garden Veggie Patties)

BEVERAGES
SUGAR-FREE DRINK MIXES:
- Crystal Light two-quart mixers
- Crystal Light Multi-Serve Bottles
- Crystal Light on the Go packets
- Crystal Light Single Serve Bottles

CARBONATED:
- Perrier Sparkling Natural Mineral Water
- Sprite Zero

CONDIMENTS/SEASONINGS/SPICES
MUSTARD
- Boar's Head Delicatessen Style Mustard

KETCHUP (Low Carb/Low Sugar)
- Heinz One Carb Reduced Sugar Tomato Ketchup

PARMESAN CHEESE (Regular or Fat Free)
- Kraft Parmesan Cheese (Original or Fat Free)

MAYONNAISE (Light/Reduced Fat/Fat Free)
- Kraft Light Mayonnaise

TOMATO SAUCE
- Hunts No Sugar Added Italian Style Sauce

IMITATION BUTTER SPRAY
- I Can't Believe It's Not Butter! Spray

NON-DAIRY CREAMER
- Nestle Coffee-mate Coffee Creamer

BALSAMIC VINEGAR
- Progresso Balsamic Vinegar

SALAD DRESSING
- Wish-Bone Salad Spritzers

WORCESTERSHIRE SAUCE
- Lea & Perrins Worcestershire Sauce

PEANUT BUTTER (Reduced Sugar, Low Sodium)
- Simply Jif Creamy Peanut Butter

NO CALORIE SWEETENER
- Splenda (Individual Packets)
- Splenda, Flavors for Coffee (Individual Sticks)

SUGAR-FREE JELLY/PRESERVES
- Smucker's Sugar Free Jam or Preserves

SUGAR-FREE SYRUP
- Vermont Sugar Free Low Calorie Syrup
- Maple Grove Farms Sugar Free Maple Flavored Syrup

ALMOND SLICES
- Sunkist Almond Accents, (Original Oven Roasted, Oven Roasted-No Salt, or Flavored)

GRANOLA
- Bear Naked Fit Granola (Vanilla Almond Crunch)

SALT-FREE SEASONING BLENDS & MARINADES
- Mrs. Dash Seasoning Blends and 10-Minute Marinades

OILS/COOKING SPRAYS
EXTRA VIRGIN OLIVE OIL
- Colavita Extra Virgin Olive Oil
- Bertoli Extra Virgin Olive Oil

CANOLA OIL
- Pure Wesson Canola Oil

Non-Stick Cooking Spray
- PAM, All Natural No-Stick Cooking Spray (Original or Flavored)

DESSERTS
SUGAR-FREE GELATIN
- Jell-O Sugar Free Low Calorie Gelatin Snacks

FAT FREE DAIRY WHIPPED TOPPING
- Reddi-wip Fat Free Dairy Whipped Topping

SUGAR-FREE POPSICLES, CREAMSICLES, FUDGSICLES
- The Original Brand, Variety Pack
- Tofutti Chocolate Fudge Treats

SUGAR-FREE GUM
- Trident Sugarless Gum

About Alison M. Fadoul

*A*lison (Ali to her friends) is a born-and-raised Floridian. Originally from Miami, her family relocated to the island of Islamorada in the heart of the Florida Keys when she was just shy of eight years old. After graduation from Coral Shores High School in 1991, she went on to attend Florida State University, earning a B.S. in criminology in 1995. Then, turning down acceptance to law school, she opted instead to attend a masters program in conflict resolution at Nova Southeastern University. In 1998, M.S. in hand, Alison left the safety bubble of school, got married, and began to explore her career options. Her path led her to enter the field of human resources.

In November 2001, Alison gave birth to a son named Mason. Holding her baby in her arms for the first time, she realized she would not be going back to the corporate world any time soon. Almost three years later, in August 2004, Alison gave birth to her second child, a daughter named Morgan. With two pregnancies under her belt, weighing twelve pounds more than she preferred at six weeks post delivery, and feeling determined to get back into shape as quickly, yet safely as possible, she caught the fitness bug—then became a SPINNING® instructor. It was during this journey that Alison experienced a moment of clarity and realized she had a calling to write a book on post-pregnancy fitness.

Ever since she was a little girl, Alison has been aware of having a purpose to contribute something meaningful. But her audience was not defined until she began her quest for health and fitness. As people began to take notice of the rewards of her eating plan and fitness regimen, they inquired about her "secrets." Alison's intention is to pay forward all she has learned and put into practice to achieve her personal best (body that is!). Her goal is to inspire other new moms to exercise and eat right so they can lose weight safely, boost their energy, and feel good about themselves and confident about their appearance.

What started out as a relatively modest project to write a short reference guide detailing the exercise program and eating plan that Alison practiced to achieve her results blossomed into a full-blown manuscript with a little help from a New York-based editor whom she gratefully stumbled upon at the right moment.

Alison and her family now reside in Miramar, Florida.

Notes

1   Tanita, "How BIA Works," http://www.tanita.com/HowBIAworks.shtml

2   U.S. Centers for Disease Control, "Body Mass Index," http://www.cdc.gov/nccdphp/dnpa/healthyweight/assessing/bmi/index.htm

3   National Heart Lung and Blood Institute, "Body Mass Index Tables" http://www.nhlbi.nih.gov/guidelines/obesity/bmi_tbl.htm

4   The International Sports Science Association, "Nutrient Ratios and Caloric Needs," http://www.bodybuilding.com/fun/issa64.htm

5   La Leche League International, "How Can I Lose Weight Safely While Breastfeeding?" http://www.llli.org/FAQ/diet.html

6   Mayo Clinic, "Dietary fats: Know which types to choose," http://mayoclinic.com/print/fat/NU00262/METHOD=print ,under subheading "Healthy fats"

7   American Heart Association, "Fats that Raise Cholesterol," http://www.americanheart.org/presenter.jhtml?identifier=4582 and "Where is saturated fat found?" http://www.nhlbi.nih.gov/health/public/heart/other/chdblack/smart1.htm

8   American Heart Association, "What Is Cholesterol?" http://www.nhlbi.nih.gov/health/dci/Diseases/Hbc/HBC_WhatIs.html

9   Mayo Clinic, "Ways to enjoy more whole grains" and "Whole grains vs. refined grains," http://www.mayoclinic.com/health/whole-grains/NU00204

10   U. S. National Library of Medicine, *Medline Plus*, "Food Sources," http://www.nlm.nih.gov/medlineplus/ency/article/002469.htm

11   U. S. National Library of Medicine, *Medline Plus*, "Food Sources," http://www.nlm.nih.gov/medlineplus/ency/article/002469.htm

12   U. S. National Library of Medicine, *Medline Plus*, "Function," http://www.nlm.nih.gov/medlineplus/ency/article/002467.htm#Function

13   U. S. National Library of Medicine, *Medline Plus*, "Recommendations," http://www.nlm.nih.gov/medlineplus/ency/article/002467.htm

14   National Cancer Institute, "Artificial Sweeteners and Cancer: Questions and Answers," http://www.cancer.gov/cancertopics/factsheet/Risk/artificial-sweeteners

The Hot Mommy Next Door

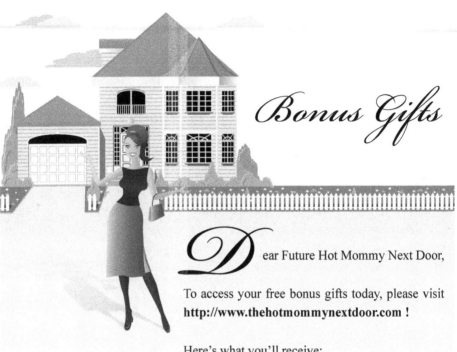

Bonus Gifts

Dear Future Hot Mommy Next Door,

To access your free bonus gifts today, please visit **http://www.thehotmommynextdoor.com** !

Here's what you'll receive:

- A list of my favorite exercises, including a special link to a website where you can view a live illustration of the exercises listed as well as execution instructions.

- A free subscription to my weekly Ezine, Tips from the Hot Mommy Next Door!

- A free audio file featuring a recorded interview with me, "America's #1 Mom Motivator" - where I discuss in detail the one-on-one consulting service I offer to get moms started on The Hot Mommy Next Door Program™!

- A free downloadable version of The Hot Mommy Next Door Shopping List featured in the book.

Health & Success,

Alison